Children and the Good Life

Children's Well-Being: Indicators and Research Series

Volume 4

Series Editor:

ASHER BEN-ARIEH

Paul Baerwald School of Social Work & Social Welfare, The Hebrew University of Jerusalem

Editorial Board:

This new series focuses on the subject of measurements and indicators of children's well being and their usage, within multiple domains and in diverse cultures. More specifically, the series seeks to present measures and data resources, analysis of data, exploration of theoretical issues, and information about the status of children, as well as the implementation of this information in policy and practice. By doing so it aims to explore how child indicators can be used to improve the development and the well being of children.

With an international perspective the series will provide a unique applied perspective, by bringing in a variety of analytical models, varied perspectives, and a variety of social policy regimes.

Children's Well-Being: Indicators and Research will be unique and exclusive in the field of measures and indicators of children's lives and will be a source of high quality, policy impact and rigorous scientific papers.

For further volumes:
http://www.springer.com/series/8162

Sabine Andresen · Isabell Diehm · Uwe Sander ·
Holger Ziegler

Editors

Children and the Good Life

New Challenges for Research on Children

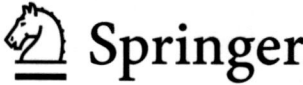 Springer

Editors
Sabine Andresen
Universität Bielefeld
Fak. Erziehungswissenschaft
Bielefeld
Germany
sabine.andresen@uni-bielefeld.de

Isabell Diehm
Universität Bielefeld
Fak. Erziehungswissenschaft
Bielefeld
Germany
isabell.diehm@uni-bielefeld.de

Uwe Sander
Universität Bielefeld
Fak. Erziehungswissenschaft
Bielefeld
Germany
uwe.sander@uni-bielefeld.de

Holger Ziegler
Universität Bielefeld
Fak. Erziehungswissenschaft
Bielefeld
Germany
holger.ziegler@uni-bielefeld.de

ISSN 1879-5196 e-ISSN 1879-520X
ISBN 978-90-481-9218-2 e-ISBN 978-90-481-9219-9
DOI 10.1007/978-90-481-9219-9
Springer Dordrecht Heidelberg London New York

Library of Congress Control Number: 2010932605

Printed on acid-free paper

Springer is part of Springer Science+Business Media (www.springer.com)

Contents

Contributors

Stefanie Albus Faculty of Educational Science, Bielefeld University, 33615 Bielefeld, Germany, stefanie.albus@uni-bielefeld.de

Sabine Andresen Faculty of Educational Science, Bielefeld University, 33615 Bielefeld, Germany, sabine.andresen@uni-bielefeld.de

Vida Beresneviciute Centre of Ethnic Studies, Institute for Social Research, Vilnius LT-08105, Lithuania, beresneviciute@ktl.mii.lt

Jérôme Ballet Center of Ethics and Economics for Environment and Development, University of Versailles Saint Quentin en Yvelines, Bd Vauban, 78047, Guyancourt, France, jballetfr@yahoo.fr

Tanja Betz German Youth Institute (DJI), 81541 Munich, Germany, betz@dji.de

Mario Biggeri Department of Economics, University of Florence, 50127 Florence, Italy, mario.biggeri@unifi.it

Zoé Clark Research School Education and Capabilities, Bielefeld University, 33615 Bielefeld, Germany, zoe.clark@uni-bielefeld.de

Tom Cockburn Department of Social Studies and Humanities, University of Bradford, Bradford BD7 1DP, UK, t.d.cockburn@bradford.ac.uk

Flavio Comim Capability and Sustainability Centre, St Edmund's College, University of Cambridge, Cambridge CB3 0BN, UK, fvc1001@cam.ac.uk

Isabell Diehm Faculty of Educational Science, Bielefeld University, 33615 Bielefeld, Germany, isabell.diehm@uni-bielefeld.de

Franziska Eisenhuth Research School Education and Capabilities, Bielefeld University, 33615 Bielefeld, Germany, franziska.eisenhuth@uni-bielefeld.de

Susann Fegter Faculty of Educational Science, Bielefeld University, 33615 Bielefeld, Germany, sfegter@uni-bielefeld.de

Didem Gürses Department of Humanities and Social Sciences, Yildiz Technical University, 34210 Esenler, Istanbul, Turkey, dgurses@yildiz.edu.tr

Akile Gürsoy Faculty of Arts and Sciences, Yeditepe University, 81120 Kayışdağı, Istanbul, Turkey, akile@yeditepe.edu.tr

Christine Hunner-Kreisel Faculty of Educational Science, Bielefeld University, 33615 Bielefeld, Germany, christine.hunner-kreisel@uni-bielefeld.de

Gonzalo Jover Faculty of Education, Complutense University of Madrid, Ciudad Universitaria, 28040 Madrid, Spain, gjover@edu.ucm.es

Tim Köhler Faculty of Educational Science, Bielefeld University, 33615 Bielefeld, Germany, tim.koehler3@uni-bielefeld.de

Melanie Kuhn Faculty of Educational Science, Bielefeld University, 33615 Bielefeld, Germany, melanie.kuhn@uni-bielefeld.de

Tadas Leončikas Centre of Ethnic Studies, Institute for Social Research, Vilnius LT-08105, Lithuania, leoncikas@ktl.mii.lt

Claudia Machold Faculty of Educational Science, Bielefeld University, 33615 Bielefeld, Germany, claudia.machold@uni-bielefeld.de

Veronika Magyar-Haas Insitute for Educational Science, Zurich University, 8032 Zurich, Switzerland, vmagyar@ife.uzh.ch

Lourdes Gaitán Muñoz Faculty of Political Science and Sociology, Complutense University of Madrid, Ciudad Universitaria, 28040 Madrid, Spain, mlourdes.gaitan@wanadoo.es

Antje Richter-Kornweitz Federal State Association for Health and Academy for Social Medicine Lower Saxony (LVGAFS), 30165 Hannover, Germany, antje.richter@gesundheit-nds.de

Martina Richter Faculty of Educational Science, Bielefeld University, 33615 Bielefeld, Germany, martina.richter1@uni-bielefeld.de

Uwe Sander Faculty of Educational Science, Bielefeld University, 33615, Bielefeld, Germany, uwe.sander@uni-bielefeld.de

Bianca Thoilliez Faculty of Education, Complutense University of Madrid, Ciudad Universitaria, 28040 Madrid, Spain, bthoilliez@edu.ucm.es

Cecile Wright School of Social Sciences, Nottingham Trent University, Nottingham, Nottinghamshire NG1 4BU, UK, cecile.wright@ntu.ac.uk

Holger Ziegler Faculty of Educational Science, Bielefeld University, 33615 Bielefeld, Germany, hziegler@uni-bielefeld.de

Introduction

Sabine Andresen, Isabell Diehm, Uwe Sander, and Holger Ziegler

In 1938, Virginia Woolf published her critical essay *Three Guineas*, in which she moved on to perform a much broader analysis of the political and cultural implications of women's oppression through inadequate education, inequality and exclusion. She pointed to the institutional and financial handicaps facing girls and women and their poverty of resources. And she was especially interested in the diversity of higher education and the achievements of formal school education. To enter the professions, she argued, women had to follow different principles. One of them is the principle of poverty as modest financial independence; another, the principle of chastity as a refusal to sell one's brain for the sake of money. From her feminist point of view, Woolf was highlighting the impact of rights, capabilities and responsibility through education. But she was also formulating the question of how education and university education need to be reformed if they are to serve as an education against war (very comprehensible in 1938). For Woolf, it was important for educational institutions to focus on the ability to empathize with others as a key competence to counter patriarchal structures.

As a feminist, Virginia Woolf was consistently trying to determine the necessary conditions for living an autonomous life. She attributed great importance to institutions such as the family and school and the latitudes that become available through access to education. Even for Woolf, it was already autonomy that was the indispensable factor for a good life, and the current discussion on the good life in general and the good life for children in particular is still concerned with the conditions and abilities that permit autonomy without ignoring dependence. As a consequence, questions on what the "good" may be and what defines a "good life" always address the image of humanity and the conditions for a fulfilling human life—what Martha Nussbaum calls "human flourishing". In the first chapter of this book, Tom Cockburn analyses this relation between autonomy and dependence, between feminist ethics and the well-being of children, that emerged in early feminist theory.

S. Andresen (✉)
Faculty of Educational Science, Bielefeld University, 33615 Bielefeld, Germany
e-mail: sabine.andresen@uni-bielefeld.de

S. Andresen et al. (eds.), *Children and the Good Life*, Children's Well-Being: Indicators and Research 4, DOI 10.1007/978-90-481-9219-9_1,
© Springer Science+Business Media B.V. 2010

Questions about children and the good life as posed in this book require not only normatively based responses, ethical reflections and sound theories but also differentiated empirical findings. When planning the present volume, we were initially guided by this tension between autonomy and dependence as a challenge to childhood studies, particularly in the field of educational science. This links up with further questions such as this: how can we simultaneously achieve both respectful caregiving *and* the freedom to choose between different options and lead a self-determined life? Or how can we link together social policies, which focus particularly on the vulnerability of children, with child-appropriate policies directed towards participation and agency? Although these are questions that may be significant for all life phases, the tensions they reflect are particularly characteristic for the life phase of childhood.

A further aspect needs to be introduced here: When we look at the major changes to the welfare state to be observed in many countries, at the problems of redistribution that have re-emerged in the international financial crisis and the fundamental changes to the environment through, for example, climate change, we can see that new questions about responsibility are being generated. The "appeal" for responsibility is an international issue on the political agenda. From the perspective of child and family policies, there is a growing need to take responsibility for all members of society, and not just for those who are actually dependent on special support or whose lives are defined by specific dependencies such as those in need of care, children, school dropouts, the unemployed, the chronically sick and the underqualified. Analyses of governmentality based on Foucault provide a critical approach with which to systematically examine the processes of exclusively privatizing responsibility. One of the things these reveal is the way in which the neoliberal discourse is always "calling" for personal responsibility.

One theory that we are working with at the *Bielefeld Centre for Education and Capability Research* and the *Research School "Education and Capability"* is that formulated by the economist Amartya Sen and the social philosopher Martha Nussbaum. This Capability Approach focuses on the latitudes of possibility and freedom and the accompanying chances that people have to realize their ability to lead a "good life". Hence, the concern is to examine which abilities, conditions and freedoms people require in order to be able to bring about this good life. This theory of justice approach, which is receiving increasing international attention, distinguishes between forms of being, known as functionings, and chances of their realization, known as capabilities. Whereas functionings focus on whether people are or do something specific, capabilities focus on the objective set of possibilities of bringing about various combinations of specific qualities of functionings. *Capabilities* are more than the possession of certain goods or the knowledge of specific cultural techniques and so forth; they are expressions of actual possibilities of being that individuals may choose "for good reasons". The Capability Approach systematically links together freedom—in the sense of social, political and cultural framing conditions—with individual abilities—in the sense of an unfolding of potentials, competencies and education. The theoretical potential of this approach lies in the development of responsibility as an issue addressing the conditions for a good life and addressing the necessary processes of negotiation to allow responsible participation for all.

This also permits what could be a new order of the social-philosophically based relation between rights and duties and the senses of responsibility for childrearing. The definition of rights and duties can and must be regulated formally through, for example, social legislation or children's rights. However, it is particularly empirical studies that show the great breadth of differences in ideas on rights and duties in daily life and the need for negotiation processes. Here as well, this addresses fundamental issues such as the following: Who is responsible to what extent for the well-being of children? Or who has the right to define and impose standards, or in what way are which groups committed to which duties? Responsibility as a relation between rights and duties can also be discussed as a question of the moral relations between parents and children or between other adults such as educators and children.

This brief sketch of our opening questions should show that the new challenges facing childhood studies do not just lie in empirical research but in nothing less than the formulation of a theory of childhood. As a theory integrating an idea of the good life, this is embedded in the traditions of social philosophy and ethics just as much as in ideas from theories of education, law and justice. We also orient ourselves towards the demand formulated by Sheila Kamerman, Shelly Phipps and Asher Ben-Arieh (2009): The knowledge generated by childhood studies and research on child indicators should be made available for policy making.

This book is based on papers presented and discussions held at a conference in Bielefeld in Spring 2009. The introductions to the single sections of the book reflect not only the state of research but also our discussions at the conference. The book is divided into four sections. It starts with the analysis of the theoretical challenges imposed by wanting to study children and their good lives. The section entitled *Children and the Good Life: Theoretical Challenges* contains chapters written by *Tanja Betz* (Munich), *Tom Cockburn* (Bradford), *Lourdes Gaitàn Muñoz* (Madrid) and *Sabine Andresen* and *Stefanie Albus* (Bielefeld). It is introduced by *Susann Fegter*, *Martina Richter* and *Claudia Machold* (all from Bielefeld) who concentrate on the new approaches and challenges to childhood studies as well as the importance of national and international social reports.

Tanja Betz discusses in her chapter conceptual and methodical reasons that favour the spread of homogenising notions about modern children and their well-being. She argues that research should reflect more the impact of unequal childhood and construct well-being from the perspective of inequality theory. *Tom Cockburn's* chapter—as mentioned above—reconstructs the phases of the discourse on the feminist ethic of care and forges systematic links to childhood studies. *Lourdes Gaitàn Muñoz* focuses on the significance of the United Nations (UN) Convention on the Rights of the Child for childhood welfare and uses her own empirical studies to discuss central issues such as cultural relativism, child labour and different degrees of responsibility. *Sabine Andresen* and *Stefanie Albus* analyse the theoretical possibilities of defining need and discuss the systematic benefits of childhood studies oriented towards need theory.

Part II, *The Capability Approach and Research on Children*, works out the significance of the Capability Approach for childhood studies and the question of the good life for children. The introduction by *Zoe Clark* and *Franziska Eisenhuth* (both from Bielefeld) analyses the potential of New Social Childhood Studies and reveals the promising ties to the capabilities perspective. The three chapters in this section link systematic theoretical concepts with their own empirical studies—an approach that promises to close gaps in research on the Capability Approach. In his chapter, *Mario Biggeri* (Florence), who works with participatory methods in his empirical studies and who has presented extremely informative empirical findings that fill out the rather vague list of the good life presented by Martha Nussbaum, addresses the impact of the Capability Approach on the field of childhood studies. *Holger Ziegler* (Bielefeld), in contrast, presents a critical analysis of the research approach to *subjective well-being* while stressing—like *Biggeri*—the potential of the Capability Approach. *Isabell Diehm* (Bielefeld) and *Veronika Magyar-Haas* (Zurich) critically discuss the one-sided perspective on language education in Germany, particularly in the German kindergarten. Based on an ethnographic study, they take a systematic approach to Nussbaum's list and the significance of literacy for children and point to different fields of language.

Part III examines *Children's Perspectives: Methodological Critique and Empirical Studies*. The introduction from *Melanie Kuhn* and *Christine Hunner-Kreisel* (both from Bielefeld) starts by examining the methodological and theoretical significance of doing research from the perspective of children. They clearly show its limitations and warn against taking a naive view of children. The three chapters from *Gonzalo Jover* and *Bianca Thoilliez* (Madrid), *Cecile Wright* (Nottingham) and *Akile Gürsoy* (Istanbul) then address specific theoretical and methodological approaches and problems. *Gonzalo Jover* and *Bianca Thoilliez* present their empirical study of children in Spain. Based on educational science, the study applies biographical theory to access the children's voice. For both authors, this is also an attempt to generate new education-based knowledge on children. *Cecile Wright* analyses the educational experiences of children in Great Britain against the background of the influence of race on their identity, social relations and agency. Theoretically, her chapter is based on concepts of ethnicity and critical discourse analyses. Particularly illuminating are her ideas on early childhood and the ability of children to reproduce dominant discourses in society. *Akile Gürsoy* looks at the development of childhood studies in Turkey. She draws on the role of the child in Turkish history, placing this in the context of the historical studies of Philippe Aries, and closes by giving examples of empirical research in Turkey and reconstructing childhood-specific topics.

Part IV completes the book with examples of *Structural Conditions and Children in Different National Contexts*. One fundamental research issue is always the relevance and weighting of specific contexts—be they either social or national. We continue to consider that social reports on national conditions, national surveys or empirical studies on special problems are indispensable. Alongside the issue of universal standards and the major significance of international comparisons, knowledge about individual contexts is also extremely important—particularly in relation to childhood and family policy. We fully endorse Alfred Kahn's insight that support for children should always be measured against one standard alone: that it should be good enough for all children (Kamerman, 2009). *Tim Köhler and Uwe Sander* (both from Bielefeld) use their introduction to examine the problems raised by the dominance of the western viewpoint and discuss criteria for making comparisons. This section contains three chapters reporting on very different countries: *Antje Richter-Kornweitz* (Hannover) on Germany, *Didem Gürses* (Istanbul) on Turkey and *Tadas Leončikas* and *Vida Beresneviciute* (Vilnius) on Lithuania. *Antje Richter-Kornweitz* performs a critical analysis of child poverty in Germany and draws conclusions for social and economic policy. She discusses poverty as a fundamental developmental risk for children in all areas of their development, and she places a particular emphasis on health. In her chapter on the well-being of children in Turkey, *Didem Gürses* reflects on the tensions between constant economic growth in recent years and the large disparities between regions and genders in terms of income distribution, health, education and political representation. She shows how this trend impacts particularly on the well-being of women and children, which groups of children are particularly exposed to poverty in Turkey, and which socio-political strategies are needed. The chapter by *Tadas Leončikas* and *Vida Beresneviciute* asks why various educational projects in Lithuania aiming at Roma integration have not succeeded in ending their exclusion. The authors present an overview of the life situation of the Roma and then analyse their position in the educational system. They point clearly to the mechanisms of exclusion and consider strategies to overcome these mechanisms.

The three final chapters in the book address children's lives in very different countries and life situations. This once again gives us an insight into how important it is to perform systematic research on different contexts and then compare political strategies and the breadth of their impact. Such research confronts the normative and universal theories for defining the good life—which have such innovative potential for childhood studies—with the necessary "irritation" of the breadth and variety of empirical findings. Nonetheless, this variety does not hide the continuous exposure to stress factors facing children and their families. Although the universality of our research questions and the Child Indicators Movement (Ben-Arieh, 2005) are confirmed by children's rights, looking both from and with the perspective of children always means taking account of the individual as well.

We received a great deal of support for our conference, and we would particularly like to thank the Rector's Office at Bielefeld University and, in particular, Martin Egelhaaf, the Prorector for Research.

The necessary editing and preparation of the present book have been generously supported by the Bielefeld Centre for Education and Capability Research. We wish to thank their speaker, Hans-Uwe Otto, and all the members of their centre. We also wish to thank our editor and translator Jonathan Harrow along with Horst Haus who was responsible for the layout. However, most of all, we wish to thank Inga Tölke. Without her tireless and competent dedication, this book would not be finished today.

Finally, we expressly thank Asher Ben-Arieh for the opportunity to publish the results of our research and discussions in the series *Children's Well-Being: Indicators and Research*. This grants us access to an excellent forum in which we can contribute to international research. Therefore, we also thank Miranda Dijksman from our publisher Springer.

References

Ben-Arieh, A. (2005). Where are the children? Children's role in measuring and monitoring their well-being. *Social Indicators Research, 74*(3), 573–596.
Kamerman, S. B. (2009). Preface. In S. B. Kamerman, S. Phipps, & A. Ben-Arieh (Eds.), *From child welfare to child well-being: An international perspective on knowledge in the service of policy making* (pp. v–x). New York: Springer.
Kamerman, S. B., Phipps, S., & Ben-Arieh, A. (Eds.). (2009). *From child welfare to child well-being: An international perspective on knowledge in the service of policy making* [Children's Well-Being: Indicators and Research Series. Vol. I]. New York: Springer.
Woolf, V. (1938/2008). *Three Guineas*. Oxford, England: Oxford University Press. (Original work published 1938)

Part I
Children and the Good Life: Theoretical Challenges

Susann Fegter, Claudia Machold, and Martina Richter

1 Introduction

Empirical research on the "good life" of children is to be found particularly under the heading "well-being," where it includes aspects of the discussion on the quality of life. There has been a marked growth in studies on childhood well-being in recent years, and they also represent an expanding field of international research. Nonetheless, they sometimes reveal major differences in how well-being is conceived. For example, studies vary greatly in the indicators they select, the ways in which these are combined, and how they are weighted (see Veenhoven, 2004). Sociological approaches to research on well-being focus more strongly on external living conditions. Nonetheless, these are assessed in a differentiated way that is not just limited to purely material aspects (see, in Germany, e.g., Bertram, 2006; Deutscher Bundestag, 2001, 2005; Hock, Holz, & Wüstendörfer, 2000; Holz, 2006; see, worldwide, e.g., Brandoli and D'Alessio, 1998, Gurses, 2006; UNICEF, 2007; Wilk, 1996). Psychological and public-health approaches, in contrast, place more emphasis on person-related indicators, and use, for example, the childhood self-concept, self-efficacy, and self-esteem as indicators of well-being (e.g., Bandura, 2006; Marks, Sha, & Westall, 2004; Pajares, 2006). Most so-called happiness research is characterized by assessing only subjective experience as an indicator of well-being and using subjective feelings of happiness or satisfaction as a measure to evaluate, for example, welfare-state provisions (e.g., Beher et al., 2007; Hascher, 2004; Hascher & Baillod, 2004; Otto & Ziegler, 2007). This has led to the criticism that such a line of research may well confuse well-being with adaptive preferences (see, on the problem of adaptive preferences, e.g., Comim, Bagolin, & Porsse, 2004). Returning to analyses of childhood well-being, more recent interdisciplinary research on poverty reveals a combination of macrostructural data

S. Fegter (✉)
Faculty of Educational Science, Bielefeld University, 33615 Bielefeld, Germany
e-mail: sfegter@uni-bielefeld.de

with subjective appraisals. This approach can be used to plot correlations between children's subjective appraisals and external conditions (see UNICEF, 2007).

Both international and German-language studies on well-being are assigning increasing importance to the viewpoints of children. These children's perspectives expand into research on well-being and are thereby leading to a reconsideration of the premises underlying contemporary childhood studies. Since the second half of the 1980s, there has been a paradigm shift in childhood research (see Grunert & Krüger, 2006; James, Jenks, & Prout, 1998; Mayall, 1994; Schweizer, 2007). In what was initially marked opposition to developmental psychology and socialization research, researchers have attempted to establish a new way of looking at children and childhood that will lead to the development of a new sociologically oriented approach addressing childhood as a social phenomenon (see Alanen, 1997; Andresen & Diehm, 2006; Lange, 2008; Qvortrup, Bardy, Sgritta, & Wintersberger, 1994; Zeiher, Büchner, & Zinnecker, 1996). What was previously often a predominantly adultist perspective directed toward developmental goals projected into the future is now being countered increasingly by a perspective focusing more strongly on the "here and now" of the child and everyday childhood life. As a result, an agent- and child-oriented research perspective in which the differences between children and adults become less important (Alanen, 1997; Qvortrup, 1987) is exerting a growing influence on the methodological debates within recent research in this field.

Both aspects mentioned above, the theoretical conceptualizations of well-being as well as the child-oriented research perspective, are currently confronting researchers with fundamental methodological and especially theoretical-normative challenges. One of these challenges is the need to consider normative postulates when defining "well-being" or the "good life." Asher Ben-Arieh (2008) has pointed out four major shifts in the field of child indicators research that deliver a deeper insight into the context of this normative issue and reveal tendencies that can be taken to be characteristic of the social studies of childhood in general. The first shift is "from survival to well-being," meaning that research interests have moved from physical survival and the basic needs of children to indicators focusing on an idea of quality of life. The second shift is summarized by "from negative to positive" and refers to a broadening of the outcomes collected to include not only negative indicators (like risk factors) but also positive ones like satisfaction. The third shift mentioned by Ben-Arieh (2008) is "from well-becoming to well-being," describing the change from a future-oriented to a present-time focus on the current well-being of the child. The fourth and last shift is called "from traditional to new domains" and refers to an extension of the field of research objects to encompass, for example, children's activities or children's friendships in order to gain a stronger child orientation. Especially the first two shifts entail a more normative and more political direction in the field of research on well-being of children, because the focus on quality of life makes stronger demands for normative decisions than research focused only on the absence of indicators causing serious harm. The more political direction can be seen clearly in the increase in policy-oriented sections within the major international surveys (see OECD, 2009; UNICEF, 2007). These studies also show that the need for normative postulates can be realized in different ways: the latest OECD Report, *Doing Better for Children* (2009), for example, refers to the UN Charter of Children's Rights when defining well-being. From the perspective of social studies of childhood, this connection is clear and convincing, because the sociological approach is closely interwoven with the children's rights movement (see Zeiher & Hengst, 2005). Other points of reference for a normative definition of the good life of children could be theories of the welfare state, medical-professional opinions, or philosophical approaches like the capability approach developed by Amartya Sen and Martha Nussbaum. The Capability Approach offers the advantage of being normative in an explicitly and theoretically reflected way (see Albus, Andresen, Fegter, & Richter, 2009). No matter which of these references is chosen, what they all share is their normativeness. We argue in favor of pointing out clearly that every conception of well-being or the good life contains a normative postulate. To avoid paternalism and an adult-oriented perspective, research projects on the good life of children should introduce participatory elements into the process of defining "the good." This leads to the second dimension of theoretical challenges.

Having said that research on well-being and children always contains normative implications regarding how well-being is defined, we now want to focus on another dimension of relevant implications and the theoretical challenges this poses. Research on well-being and children does not just constitute its object of research (well-being) in a normative sense; it is also based on assumptions about its research subject (children). This aspect reveals the need for a broader reflection on the constructions of difference within this research. We assume that childhood and children cannot be understood as an anthropological constant but rather as a socially and historically constructed stage of human life. Throughout history, the first years of human life have been conceived very differently. One example of this is to be found in Philipp Ariès's (1962) *Centuries of Childhood*, in which he claims that the idea of childhood did not even exist in medieval society. Hence, ideas on and concepts of children have to be understood within their sociohistorical context. This makes it necessary to ask which ideas have dominated the way children are defined in recent times. Research and theory formulation can be seen as part of the production of certain knowledge about children. The change of paradigm within childhood studies mentioned above has taken this into account, and the sociology of childhood delivered an important impulse to the way children are seen within research. Its notion of children as social actors challenged the idea of dependent and developing children. Methodologically, this is expressed by the shift from research *on children* to research *with children* or even *from the perspective of children*. Thus, the change of paradigm also implies a change in the conceptualization of the research subject children. Although deconstructive childhood studies now acknowledge this fundamental shift, they point to the attendant risk of romanticizing children and misconceiving their dependence within the social order of society. Therefore, it is necessary to stress that reflection on the ideas produced about children not only is an important end in itself but is also important from an *ethical* point of view. With regard to Alanen's (2001, 2005) concept of "generationing," one can say that the way children are constructed within a certain sociohistorical context is fundamentally linked to power relations. She understands generation as a social structure that regulates the relation between the groups involved. This social order does not exist per se, but is reproduced in social practice. Generation as a relational structure determines the power, recourses, and possibilities of participation available to social actors. With reference to children and adults, it can be assumed that children are the powerless group lacking any possibilities of participation. Furthermore, the notion of children has to be seen in terms of its differentiation from adults and in the way it is constructed in social processes. One element is the permanent "othering" of children that takes place every time *we* talk, write, and do research about *them*. This becomes an ethical concern insofar as research from this perspective is involved in processes of "generationing" and therefore in the (re-)production of power relations. This is also a concern for research into the well-being of children and the question raised above on the normative decisions made in relation to the conceptualization of well-being. When deciding from a researcher's point of view what we understand as "the good" *for* children, we always produce a generational difference. At the same time, this insight enables us to analyze the theories of well-being in terms of how they articulate and reproduce the generational order.

As a consequence, it becomes necessary to reflect on the ideas (re-)produced, either explicitly or implicitly, within the theoretical assumptions underlying research into children, and to question what othering is taking place and which effects this has on processes of generationing. Moreover, these questions do not just arise in respect to generation. They can just as similarly be reflected in other differences: What assumptions about class, gender, or ethnicity underlie the research design?

Nonetheless, having stressed the deconstructive perspective on childhood studies, we should not forget the other side of the coin and the other ethical dimension it raises: Although research on children (re-)produces certain notions about children, it does, at the same time, still give voice to this marginalized group.

To conclude, we would like to emphasize that no matter which theoretical assumptions (feminist care, children's rights) are made either implicitly or explicitly, research has to be aware of its normative impact on society and its subjectivity— be it in terms of either the idea of "the good" or the social order of generation. At the same time, it remains a necessary way to give voice to children, or at least to cast light on the needs of those marginalized within the generational relation. The following authors have responded to these challenges in very productive and interesting ways.

References

Alanen, L. (1997). Soziologie der Kindheit als Projekt: Perspektiven für die Forschung. *Zeitschrift für Sozialisationsforschung und Erziehungssoziologie, 17*(2), 162–178.
Alanen, L. (2001). Childhood as a generational condition: Children's daily lives in a central Finland town. In L. Alanen & B. Mayall (Eds.), *Conceptualising child-adult relations* (pp. 129–153). London: Routledge Falmer.
Alanen, L. (2005). Kindheit als generationales Konzept. In H. Hengst & H. Zeiher (Eds.), *Kindheit soziologisch* (pp. 65–81). Wiesbaden: VS-Verlag.

Albus, S., Andresen, S., Fegter, S., & Richter, M. (2009). Wohlergehen und das "gute Leben" in der Perspektive von Kindern. Das Potenzial des Capability Approach für die Kindheitsforschung. *Zeitschrift für Soziologie der Erziehung und Sozialisation. Schwerpunktheft Capability Forschung, 29*(4), 346–358.

Andresen, S., & Diehm, I. (Eds.). (2006). *Kinder, Kindheiten, Konstruktionen.* Wiesbaden: VS-Verlag.

Ariès, P. (1962). *Centuries of childhood: A social history of family life* (R. Baldick, Trans.). New York: Knopf.

Bandura, A. (2006). Adolescent development from an agentic perspective. In F. Pajares & T. Urdan (Eds.), *Self-efficacy beliefs of adolescents* (pp. 1–43). Greenwich, CT: Information Age Publishing.

Beher, K., Haenisch, H., Hermens, C., Nordt, G., Prein, G., & Schulz, U. (2007). *Die offene Ganztagsschule in der Entwicklung. Empirische Befunde zum Primarbereich in Nordrhein-Westfalen.* Weinheim/Munich: Juventa.

Ben-Arieh, A. (2008). The child indicators movement: Past, present, and future. *Child Indicator Research, 1,* 3–16.

Bertram, H. (2006). *Zur Lage der Kinder in Deutschland: Politik für Kinder als Zukunftsgestaltung.* (Innocenti Working Paper No. 2006-02). Florence, Italy: UNICEF Innocenti Research Centre.

Brandolini, A., & D'Alessio, G. (1998). *Measuring well-being in the functioning space.* Rome: Banca d'Italia.

Comim, F., Bagolin, I., & Porsse, M. (2004). Adaptive preferences: A problem or a good guide? Paper at the The 4th International Conference on the Capability Approach: Enhancing Human Security 5–7 September 2004–University of Pavia, Italy http://www-3.unipv.it/deontica/ca2004/papers/bagolin%20porsse%20comim.pdf

Deutscher Bundestag. (2001). *Lebenslagen in Deutschland. Erster Armuts- und Reichtumsbericht.* (Drucksache 14/15990). Berlin: Deutscher Bundestag.

Deutscher Bundestag. (2005). *Lebenslagen in Deutschland. Zweiter Armuts- und Reichtumsbericht.* (Drucksache 15/5015). Berlin: Deutscher Bundestag.

Grunert, C., & Krüger, H. (2006). *Kindheit und Kindheitsforschung in Deutschland. Forschungszugänge und Lebenslagen.* Opladen: Barbara Budrich.

Gurses, D. (2006). *Development of a comprehensive policy to fight child poverty in Turkey.* Paper presented at the International Conference of the Human Development and Capability Association, Groningen, Netherlands. Accessed December 28, 2009, from http://capabilityapproach.com/pubs/6_4_Gurses.pdf

Hascher, T. (2004). *Wohlbefinden in der Schule.* Münster: Waxmann.

Hascher, T., & Baillod, J. (2004). Soziale Integration in der Schulklasse als Prädiktor für Wohlbefinden. In T. Hascher (Ed.), *Schule positiv erleben* (pp. 133–160). Bern: Haupt.

Hock, B., Holz, G., & Wüstendörfer, W. (2000). *"Frühe Folgen – Langfristige Konsequenzen?" Armut und Benachteiligung im Vorschulalter. Vierter Zwischenbericht zu einer Studie im Auftrag des Bundesverbandes der Arbeiterwohlfahrt.* Frankfurt a. M.: ISS.

Holz, G. (2006). *"Zukunftschancen für Kinder!?" – Wirkung von Armut bis zum Ende der Grundschulzeit. Endbericht der 3. AWO-ISS-Studie im Auftrag der Arbeiterwohlfahrt Bundesverband e.V.* Frankfurt a. M.: ISS. Accessed December 28, 2009, from http://www.unipv. it/deontica/ca2004/papers/bagolin%20porsse%20comim.pdf

James, A., Jenks, C., & Prout, A. (1998). *Theorizing childhood.* Cambridge: Polity.

Lange, A. (2008). Soziologie der Kindheit und frühkindliche Bildung. In W. Thole, H.-G. Rossbach, M. Fölling-Albers, & R. Tippelt (Eds.), *Bildung und Kindheit. Pädagogik der frühen Kindheit in Wissenschaft und Lehre* (pp. 65–81). Opladen: Barbara Budrich.

Marks, N., Sha, H., & Westall, A. (2004). *The power and potential of well-being indicators. Measuring young people's well-being in Nottingham.* London: NEF.

Mayall, B. (Ed.). (1994). *Children's childhoods observed and experienced.* London: Routledge Falmer.

OECD (2009). *Doing better for children.* Paris: Author.

Otto, H.-U., & Ziegler, H. (2007). Soziale Arbeit, Glück und das gute Leben. In S. Andresen, I. Pinhard, & S. Weyers (Eds.), *Erziehung – Ethik – Erinnerung* (pp. 229–248). Weinheim: Beltz.

Pajares, F. (2006). Self-efficacy during childhood and adolescence. Implications for teachers and parents. In F. Pajares & T. Urban (Eds.), *Self-efficacy beliefs of adolescents* (pp. 339–367). Greenwich, CT: Information Age Publishing.

Qvortrup, J. (1987). Introduction. *International Journal of Sociology, Special Issue: The Sociology of Childhood, 17*(3), 3–37.

Qvortrup, J., Bardy, M., Sgritta, G., & Wintersberger, H. (Eds.) (1994). *Childhood matters. Social theory, practice and politics*. Aldershot: Avebury.

Schweizer, H. (2007). *Soziologie der Kindheit. Verletzlicher Eigen-Sinn*. Wiesbaden: VS-Verlag.

UNICEF. (2007). *Child poverty in perspective: An overview of child well-being in rich countries*. (Innocenti Report Card 7). Florence: UNICEF Innocenti Research Centre.

Veenhoven, R. (2004). *Subjective measures of well-being*. (Discussion Paper No. 2004/07). Helsinki: UNU-Wider. Accessed December 28, 2009, from http://www.wider.unu.edu/ publications/working-papers/discussion-papers/2004/en_GB/dp2004-007/

Wilk, L. (1996). Die Studie "Kindsein in Österreich". Kinder und ihre Lebenswelten als Gegenstand empirischer Sozialforschung – Chancen und Grenzen einer Surveyerhebung. In M.-S. Honig (Ed.), *Kinder und Kindheit: soziokulturelle Muster – sozialisationstheoretische Perspektiven* (pp. 55–76). Weinheim: Juventa.

Zeiher, H., Büchner, P., & Zinnecker, J. (Eds.) (1996). *Kinder als Außenseiter? Umbrüche in der gesellschaftlichen Wahrnehmung von Kindern und Kindheit*. Munich: Juventa.

Zeiher, H., & Hengst, H. (2005). Von Kinderwissenschaften zu generationalen Analysen. Einleitung. In H. Zeiher & H. Hengst (Eds.), *Kindheit soziologisch* (pp. 9–24). Wiesbaden: VS-Verlag.

Modern Children and Their Well-Being: Dismantling an Ideal

Tanja Betz

Childhood is a culturally formed and socially constructed concept that is subject to constant change. This becomes clear in the changeable, yet persevering institutionalized hierarchy between adults and children spanning multiple aspects of society—a hierarchy regulated by law in child protection or child welfare domains inter alia (Mierendorff, 2008) and coupled with its own respective child and youth welfare policy.

Hence, childhood must always be viewed in the context of social change; the concept of a "good childhood" is closely linked to changeable cultural, social and economic circumstances (Bühler-Niederberger & van Krieken, 2008; Kränzl-Nagl & Mierendorff, 2008; Qvortrup, 2005). Likewise, societal changes and modernization spurts affect the concrete shaping of children's lives (Fölling-Albers et al., 2005).

A modernization theoretical research field that deals with these change processes and their effects on children's lives has emerged in childhood research (Dencik, 1995; Roppelt, 2003).[1] Within this field of research, but also well beyond in policy and practice, the modernization process is associated with various societal changes that flow into the description of modern children and their lives.

Frequently, in this context, a picture is painted that implies intergenerational relations are less hierarchically structured today than they were in the past. Accordingly, modern childhood patterns in the family are presented as a result of the transformation of the so-called command households into negotiation households—a transition that goes hand in hand with the shift of the parent-figure away from the unapproachable authority person towards that of an advisor or conversation and negotiation partner for the child (du Bois-Reymond, 2005). The interaction forms in (modern) families are characterized by symmetry and reasoning (Wild, 2004). Parents perceive their children as individuals in their own right (Dencik, 1995); the pillars of

---

T. Betz (✉)
German Youth Institute (DJI), 81541 Munich, Germany
e-mail: betz@dji.de

[1] Similar research fields pertaining to modernization theory can also be found in youth research (Gille, Sardei-Biermann, Gaiser, & de Rijke, 2006).

S. Andresen et al. (eds.), *Children and the Good Life*, Children's Well-Being: Indicators and Research 4, DOI 10.1007/978-90-481-9219-9_2,
© Springer Science+Business Media B.V. 2010

modernized parent-child relationships are the limited application of parental punishment and great respect for children's interests (Kötters, 2000). Parents emphasize
the autonomy, cooperation ability and creativity of their children; they have replaced
the norms and rearing goals of the past based on discipline, order and obedience
(Fölling-Albers et al., 2005). The thesis of the modern negotiation household[2] is
finding broad acceptance; the empirical findings are seen as "the current state of
contemporary German childhood"[3] (Honig, 1999, p. 158).

There are further indicators that flow into the description of the current shaping
of children's lives. For instance, both modern mothers and modern fathers are seen
as predominantly employed. They deal with the education and supervision of their
children, who in turn spend their time in facilities of the public day-care and education systems (keyword: "cared childhood"; Dencik, 1995). Moreover, parents are
described as being interested in the academic progress of their children; they expect
high educational qualifications (Fölling-Albers et al., 2005) and are very much willing to contribute to academic commitment (Wild, 2004). Modern children have at
their disposal their own rooms in the household—not only for completing homework assignments. Last but not least, as in the past, the predominant modern family
is seen as a father-mother-child family, although other family forms are also gaining
acceptance (Fölling-Albers et al., 2005).

The modern childhood pattern can also be identified, so the general tenor, in
leisure contexts. For instance, Fuhs (2002) states that modern childhood is a "club
childhood", i.e. it is planned and organized, and children spend their "free" time
primarily in clubs and associations. Sports clubs, in particular, are very popular in
this context ("over-sported childhood"). Correspondingly, modern childhood is also
described as a "scheduled childhood": Clubs, as well as other leisure time facilities
or special tuition, are replacing "free" time in favour of strictly scheduled events
with fixed timetables geared towards (early) advancement. The media, other authors
find, also play an important role in the life of the modern child; referred to as the
so-called "mediatized childhood". Cell phones, text messages, e-mail, the Internet,
computer games and game consoles are "matter-of-course in children's everyday
world" (Ministerium für Schule & Jugend und Kinder (MSJK), 2005, p. 35).

These phenomena, which are only briefly described here, seem to be synonyms
for a modern childhood pattern; the requisite data is often interpreted as if it were
equally valid for all children today. Further diagnoses are mostly added to these
descriptions: "certain levelling tendencies within the childhood population" have
been diagnosed; childhoods "are becoming increasingly homogenous" in comparison to the past, with large class-specific differences losing relevance (Kränzl-Nagl &
Mierendorff, 2008, p. 10ff.). In short, the modern child is part of a child group
that is relatively homogenous but in no way characterized by social class. Also, in
internationally oriented surveys different elements of the living conditions of "the"

---

[2] This thesis can mainly be traced back to the international project "Modernisierung von Kindheit"
(Modernization of childhood) (du Bois-Reymond et al., 1994).

[3] Most citations in this paper stem from German sources and have been translated into English.

contemporary children are collected, average values determined, indices set up and different aspects of the well-being of children in various countries compared and contrasted (Bertram & Kohl, 2010; OECD, 2009; UNICEF, 2007).

There is however, and hence this chapter, room for doubt as to whether the findings behind the modernization theory are sustainable and do indeed grant accurate insights into contemporary children's lives. When analyzing recent large-scale, Germany-wide studies, the so-called children's surveys from a theoretical perspective of inequality, there is hardly any empirical evidence for the prevalent perceptions. However, conceptual as well as methodical reasons can be discerned that favour the spread of homogenizing notions about modern children and their well-being. Given the aforementioned research perspective, it does, nonetheless, appear more appropriate to talk about "unequal childhoods" and therefore to consistently disaggregate the children's group conceptually as well as in empirical analysis according to the factors gender, milieu/class and ethnicity.[4] At the same time, there is one finding that seems paradoxical at first sight, namely that nearly independently of "real" conditions of inequality, almost all children state that they feel good in their family and at school. That is why the construct "well-being", which is widespread in children's surveys and international comparative studies working with self-reports, should be challenged.

After a brief introduction to children's surveys (1) this chapter will examine how far the widespread notions of the modern child are indeed supported by current empirical findings about children's lives (2) and what basis there is for the spread of the homogenous modernization findings. (3) The construct "well-being" is then analyzed in more detail and reinterpreted from the perspective of inequality theory. (4) An outlook (5) calls for a continuous verification of the modernization diagnoses and a reflection on the implications of the prevalent perceptions.

1 The Data Source: Children's Surveys

As instruments of continuous monitoring of societal processes and structures, social reporting and its subdomain of children's surveys (Betz, 2008) aim at analyzing socio-structural changes (Noll, 2004). These can be observed via the empirical analysis of the modernization process, including its problems, prerequisites, consequences and implications. Aside from official data, elements of social change and its implications for children can be documented with standardized children's surveys, i.e. indicator-based questionnaires for children as of the age of approximately 6 years (and their parents), on current conditions of growing up and children's lives from a children's perspective. In this way, both the general population and policy makers, as well as practicing professionals in the field and in research can gain

---

[4]There are further, similarly important, differentiation factors for the adequate description of the children's life and living conditions such as "region" and "country", which cannot be addressed in more detail here.

insights into the living conditions of modern children. The aim is to describe child-hood using meaningful indicators. At the same time, this data can be used to reassess popular modernization diagnoses. The representative design will help to ensure that all child groups are given equal opportunities for the living conditions, attitudes and behaviour patterns typical of "their" life to become a part of the description of modern childhood patterns.

2 The Findings: Migration Background, Social Class and Gender Shape Childhood

Three exemplary areas of children's lives that have become central elements in the description of the modern child will be elaborated on by drawing on the findings of two representative German children's surveys. On the one hand, findings from the German Youth Institute's Children's Panel will be used (Alt, 2005; Betz, 2008), a longitudinal children's survey begun in 2002 that contains inter alia direct interviews of 8–9-year-olds and their parents. On the other hand the findings of the first World Vision Children's Study will be reported—a cross-sectional, pure children's survey with 8–11-year-old children that was launched in 2007[5] (World Vision Deutschland e. V. (WVD), 2007).

Based on these surveys, the term "equal rights negotiation household" can be broken down using example of indicators for pocket money allocation in the family, for disputes about money between parents and children and for forms and frequency of parental punishment for the surveyed children. Overall 51% of the 8–9-year-olds receive pocket money regularly, 22% receive no pocket money, 27% irregularly. Gender differences are small: Girls tend to get pocket money more seldom than boys (WVD, 2007, p. 99ff.). Class differences, on the other hand, are more obvious: 35% of lower-class children receive pocket money regularly, as opposed to 77% of the children from higher classes, which corresponds to a 2.2-fold difference. The differ-ences between children with or without migration background are smaller, they do however point in the same general direction: 46% of the children with a migration background receive a regular allowance, while for native German children the num-ber is 61%, i.e. 1.3 times higher (ibid.). Overall, among the 8–9-year-old children money-related family conflicts between parents and children only take place "now and again". Here, there are no differences, neither between genders, nor between milieus or ethnic groups (Betz, 2008, p. 261ff.).

When asked about punishments, children indicate that "talking without punish-ment" (WVD, 2007, p. 102ff.) is usual when the parents are angry with the children

---

[5]The questionnaires from both studies are available online or in the respective publications; the basic design of the studies is described in Table 1. A third, also Germany-wide study, the "LBS Children's Barometer Germany 2009" (LBS-Initiative Junge Familie, 2009), cannot be considered here, as the findings from $N = 10,194$ children between 9 and 14 years have not been compiled with sufficient differentiation and the class/milieu affiliation of the children was not covered.

(boys: 81%; girls: 80%). Nevertheless, "scolding" is common (boys: 79%; girls: 71%), followed by "forbidding things" (boys: 68%; girls: 55%) and "cutting pocket money" (boys: 14%; girls: 8%). Children also report forms of parental violence (slaps in the face/beating), albeit these are by far less common (boys: 19%; girls: 10%). Class differences in terms of punishments are not differentiated in the study; parental violence is most common in lower classes, in particular with regard to sons.

A further diagnosis in the modernization discourse, the "mediatized childhood," can be verified using recent indicators for computer use, internet access and internet use. It turns out that 74% of the 8–9-year-old children use a computer (Betz, 2008, p. 273ff.); boys (78%) more frequently than girls (69%). Moreover, social differences are significant: While 61% of the children from milieus with limited resources use a computer, there are 83% computer users among children from well-off milieus (ibid.). Native children have the highest rate of computer use and children of Turkish origin the lowest, while children of Russian origin take a middle position (ibid., p. 344ff.). Although smaller, the correlation with internet access is similar: 54% of the 8–11-year old girls and boys have access to the Internet; 21% of them are online regularly and here, too, there are as good as no gender differences (WVD, 2007, p. 188ff.). However, 26% of the lower-class children have internet access compared with 66% of the higher-class children, a 2.5 times higher rate. A significantly lower correlation is displayed when comparing children with and without migration background. While only 43% of the former have internet access at their disposal, the rate for native children is 1.3 times higher at 57% (ibid.).

As to the established diagnosis of the modern "club childhood", current data on club involvement shows that 58% of the 8–9-year-old girls and boys participate in a club (Betz, 2008). There are significant differences between children from different milieus: 34% of the children from a nonprivileged milieu, as opposed to 78% of the children from the milieu with the most extensive resources, are active in clubs, i.e. more than 2.2 times as many (ibid., p. 279ff.). Overall the involvement in sports clubs is most frequent (85%), with clear differences according to gender: 44% of the girls and 56% of the boys do sports (ibid., WVD, 2007). Moreover, club involvement is least characteristic for the life situation of children of Turkish and Russian origin from milieus with lower resources: around one quarter of them is involved in clubs;[6] for the corresponding native children group that number is 61%, which represents a 2.4 times higher rate (Betz, 2008, p. 351).

These results alone suffice to make three points clear. First of all, they illustrate that "the societal modernization spurt affects milieu-specific children groups in different ways" (Fölling-Albers et al., 2005, p. 160f.), just as with children of different ethnicity, and that there are "non-synchronisms in societal shift in nearly all areas", so that not all children are affected in the same way by economic, cultural or social changes (ibid.). Hence, both aspects of childhood characterized as

---

[6]Twenty four percentage of the children of Turkish origin participate in a club and 25% in the group with Russian origin (ibid.).

traditional and those characterized as modern occur simultaneously (Roppelt, 2003; Zinnecker, 2001).

Second, it becomes obvious that the assumption of the growing irrelevance of the class/milieu category in describing children's lives and the widespread descriptions of a prevalently homogenous child population are hardly sustainable. The designation "club children", for instance, can be used to accurately label just over a third of the children from nonprivileged milieus and only about a quarter of the children from families of Turkish or Russian origin. And although over time the rates of club involvement have risen, the number of personal computers (PCs) in the families has grown and parental punishment in child rearing has declined, the differences within child groups have not disappeared. Yet the established descriptions, including political ones, create notions and perceptions of a fictive, average modern child (cf. Chapter 5).

Third, the demonstrated differences between children are in no way merely an expression of heterogeneous lives of children. They are rather an indicator of unequal opportunities to partake in relevant social commodities. For instance, the experience and knowledge involved in dealing with computers, the activity in (sports) clubs or the regular handling of (pocket) money represent expectations that, among other things, can be asked for and rewarded by teachers at school.

3 The Shortcomings: Concept and Method Distort the Picture

There are certainly many answers to the question of why social and ethnic differences, in particular, in the living conditions of children are not the subject of childhood studies and why inequalities are not exposed or, as James and James (2004) ask, why "even within societies, the diversities in children's experiences are often masked, downplayed (...) for the sake of emphasising commonality?" (ibid., p. 30). Some of the reasons for the construction of a homogenous child group in childhood research can be traced back to the conceptual and empirical level. However, this by no means extends to a child group disaggregated according to the sociologically common factors of social inequality such as class/milieu.

The analysis of social and ethnic differentiation factors within the child group is conceptually undesirable. Many authors say, childhood is to be treated as a uniform phenomenon; children allegedly have more in common than they do not, and that should also be made clear in research access (e.g. Qvortrup, 2005). Analyses of childhoods that are class-specific and vary according to ethnic groups, or also those of gender-typical patterns of childhood should not be seen as childhood studies per se, but respectively class, migration or gender studies (ibid.). Independent of their differentiation in subgroups, children should be analyzed in their quality as children confronted with specific development tasks. These arguments presented here only briefly can be traced back to the establishment of the "New Sociology of Childhood". The formation of Childhood Studies and their analogies to Women's Studies (Alanen, 2002) is probably to blame for the fact that the "gender" dimension plays a much more central role in the analyses, both conceptually and empirically, than "milieu/class" or "ethnicity" (see below). The generation axis is perceived as the central inequality axis. Other, in part transverse, inequality axes stand behind.

Reasons for the neglect of specific differences based on ethnicity and milieu/class within the child group can also be found at the empirical level. By analyzing children's surveys (Betz, 2009) or also during careful examinations of international comparative studies, it can be clearly demonstrated how a homogenous modern child group is constructed, namely by omitting or only partially taking into account the internal differentiation of the overall group of children—especially in international comparative studies also according to age—in spite of the fact that the survey sample size would have allowed for such differentiation. The latter applies at the very least to children from different social milieus. That is not the case for descriptions of childhoods of different groups with a migration background: These cannot yet be represented with the current survey sample sizes (for Germany: Betz, 2009). A further factor is the incomplete data pool, which does not permit analyses of subgroups (a showcase example being the OECD study "Doing better for children": OECD, 2009). Alone the fact that up to 2010 no solid, extensible and disaggregatable data stock was built up can be viewed as a clear indication that the institutionalized hierarchy between adults and children is proving to be a very robust societal power structure over time.

An exact analysis of older children's surveys in Germany from the years 1980/1990 (Betz, 2008, 2009) shows that there are differences in children's lives, in particular, according to age groups and school forms. Yet, different populations and child groups are targeted, depending on the sample design. Systematic distortions can be identified to the disadvantage of special needs students, who are for the most part excluded. Moreover, it can be shown that there is a greater interest to describe the living conditions and the quality of life of boys and girls. More in-depth differentiations of the child group and the description of "unequal childhoods" in terms of social class and ethnicity seem less relevant.

In more recent children's surveys starting in the year 2000, there are both changes and constancy (see Table 1; Betz, 2009).

The recourse to a school sample (e.g. LBS-Initiative Junge Familie, 2009) still means that special needs students are omitted; the social affiliation of children is not consistently relevant (ibid.). Ethnic affiliation has become more significant; however children are mostly divided into two large groups: children with and without a migration background. This does not do justice to the internal differentiation of both groups, especially with view to circumstances of inequality (review: Betz, 2008) or also regarding self-attributions and placements (Hamburger & Stauf, 2009). The "gender" category, on the other hand, is consistently given relevance.

The fact is, that those subpopulations of the child group that can be reached easily using standardized research methods—and this is also true for adult populations—are given priority. Because of the minor importance given to the aforementioned differentiation criteria, also conceptually, the child group appears as a single large group, but in any case not as an unequal child group.

Table 1 Germany-wide representative and differentiated children's surveys since 2000

Children's surveys

DJI Children's Panel (Alt, 2005; Betz, 2008)
$N = 1,561$
Age group: children between 8 and 9 years
Longitudinal study: 1st wave in 2002
Sampling concept: Child sample
Differentiation criteria:
Gender: Relevant
Social affiliation (social class and milieu): Relevant
Ethnic affiliation: Relevant
Based on threefold migration concept
(children of Turkish origin, of Russian origin, native German children)

1*st World Vision Children's Study* (World Vision Deutschland e. V., 2007)
$N = 1,592$
Age group: children between 8 and 11 years
Cross-section Study in 2007
Sampling concept: Child sample
Differentiation criteria:
Gender: Relevant
Social affiliation (social class): Relevant
Ethnic affiliation: Relevant
Based on a dichotomous migration concept
(children with/without migration background)

Source: compiled by the author

Empirical evidence also suggests that a general underrepresentation of children with a migration background, as well as children from lower social classes can be assumed; children attending special needs schools are also often not included. The specifics of the latter child group—which, once again, many children with a migration background belong to—have a very low chance of even finding their way into the common descriptions of the lives of modern children; the same applies to children of refugees and asylum seekers. German or German-speaking children from the middle classes, on the other hand, are much more likely to leave their mark on prevalent perceptions. An analysis of the living conditions of children from various immigrant groups and children from precarious social milieus, on the other hand, are often given marginal notice only.[7] The living conditions of the average modern child are thus constructed, intentionally or otherwise, via conceptual assumptions, study design and the interpretation of the findings.

It is, however, also not possible to empirically base the idea of "new" dissimilar childhoods on the findings of the children's surveys (Bühler-Niederberger, 2009).

---

[7]Omitted here are further details with research relevance such as the selection of indicators or the intention of the questions. There is evidence that many questions in the children's surveys are targeted at the high culture practices of middle class children (Betz, 2008).

For empirical evidence proving that childhoods are becoming more unequal one would need longitudinal data and long-term studies—like those conducted in child poverty or education research, for example—as well as long-term monitoring or social reporting on children that is not just propagated, but also implemented. These kinds of studies and monitoring are as of yet nonexistent in German-speaking countries. The diversity in the sampling concept, the age groups respectively included in the studies (cf. Table 1), as well as the various indicators, approaches and (policy) objectives make a chronological comparative analysis difficult.

Instead of institutionalized permanent monitoring of the living conditions and well-being of children, the popularity of certain topics, which are then followed by scientific discourses, draws attention to specific notions of childhood, as well as specific categories and classifications (Kränzl-Nagl & Mierendorff, 2008). This is done without sufficient scientific deliberation.

So one can conclude, based on existing children's surveys and studies of childhood—so far at least—social change is less discernable than changes in empirical approaches to children and childhood, thematic priorities and the respective underlying concepts and variable policy goals. Only in recent years have unequal childhoods started to receive greater attention in childhood research (Betz, 2008, 2009).

4 Monitoring Child Well-Being: Possibilities and Limitations

In nearly all children's surveys the "well-being" construct plays a central role. In this context it stands primarily for the "subjective experience" of "objective living conditions" (Bertram, 2008; Wilk & Bacher, 1994).[8] Information about well-being is obtained predominantly from children themselves, the parents are only rarely asked to provide information to this end (exemplary findings in Betz, 2008). Child well-being is determined directly via specific indicators ("How well do you feel in your family/at school?") or indirectly, for instance as an element of the family climate. The values are then analyzed separately by indicator, but most of them are also aggregated across different areas (LBS-Initiative Junge Familie, 2009; WVD, 2007). Depending on the exact wording of the question(s), the compilation of the well-being index and its aggregation level or the respective weighting of the individual indicators and further factors, a wide range of findings ensues, thus making comparability—in particular with the international research on the well-being of children (see below)—nearly impossible.

---

[8]There is a wide range of ideas and concepts on the well-being of children and on their measurement using standardized indicators. The respective concepts cannot be discussed and contrasted here in more detail (revealing: Ben-Arieh, 2008; Bradshaw, Hoelscher, & Richardson, 2007; OECD, 2009; UNICEF, 2007).

German studies based on self-reports of children, however, indicate concordantly that the prevailing majority of children today feel (very) good: 88% of the 8–11-year-olds make this claim (WVD, 2007, p. 220ff.). At the same time, children predominantly feel better in their family than at school, although here, too, the values are high. Overall, boys feel a somewhat lower level of well-being than girls (ibid.; Betz, 2008, p. 254ff.).

The findings on ethnic affiliation, on the other hand, are not conclusive: It has been proven that migration background has no effect on the well-being of children (WVD, 2007, p. 224). When using other data sets, however, especially for children of Turkish origin, there is evidence for much higher rates of (family) well-being (Betz, 2008, p. 329f., p. 353ff.). The findings pertaining to the relevance of the category milieu/class are also inconsistent. While one study shows a level of lower well-being merely for lower-class children (WVD, 2007, p. 223f.), results based on different data show small to no differences between children from different milieus regarding school well-being (Betz, 2008, p. 287) and no differences regarding family well-being (ibid., p. 254f.). Consequently nearly all children feel (very) good and are satisfied.

At an international level, too, a wide field of research on the well-being of children has emerged (Ben-Arieh, 2008; Bradshaw, Hoelscher, & Richardson, 2006). The OECD for instance has established a multidimensional monitoring system for child well-being, which includes an international comparison of OECD countries in six dimensions. These include material well-being, housing and environment, educational well-being, health, risk behaviours, and quality of school life (OECD, 2009), and are each mapped via multiple indicators. Questions on the subjective well-being of children, common in German children's surveys, are not included. The argument for this is that the monitoring system and, respectively, the international report have a strong policy focus and "it is unclear how governments concerned with (. . .) subjective well-being would go about designing policies to improve outcomes (in this dimension)" (ibid., p. 29; elision and insertion T. B.).[9]

Furthermore, a monitoring system for the well-being of children in African countries, which is in turn different from the OECD and also from the UNICEF (see below) surveys, was recently put into place (African Child Policy Forum, 2008). For the African continent, a so-called child-friendliness index is calculated based on two dimensions, "provision" and "protection", which in turn—similar to OECD and UNICEF—are compiled from various indicators. This index is meant to show, among other things, how far African countries ensure the well-being of children. Also, this monitoring system geared towards the well-being of children does not include the subjective well-being of children. The argument is the lack of national data—the same problem applies to the plan to include "participation" empirically as a third conceptual dimension in this reporting system. Here, data is also not available (ibid., p. 41).

---

[9]Using the same argumentation, "family and peer relationships" play no role in the OECD monitoring, in contrast to UNICEF (OECD, 2009).

UNICEF has also set up transnational monitoring for the well-being of children of (not only) OECD countries (UNICEF, 2007; but also on the situation of children in Germany: Bertram, 2006; Bertram & Kohl, 2010). Here, too, child well-being is more broadly defined and empirically recorded than in German children's surveys; it covers six dimensions, four of which are effectively the same as in the OECD system. In an international comparison the dimensions of family and peer relationships, behaviours and risks, health and safety, as well as school, material and subjective well-being are mapped and contrasted using a number of indicators (UNICEF, 2007). Subjective well-being is, in turn, subdivided into three equally weighted dimensions (Bertram, 2008, p. 77ff.; UNICEF, 2007, p. 35ff.).[10]

Interestingly, the subjective well-being dimension here is comparable to the concepts in children's surveys in Germany. As such, comparisons between the different studies can be made. However, while the children in the UNICEF study are in part differentiated according to age group and gender, distinctions by ethnic groups or social milieu are not made. Hence, a sufficient disaggregation of the findings is not possible.

Regarding the subjective assessment of one's own personal well-being, the UNICEF study establishes a cumulative value for Germany. The rates of well-being for Germany are high, placing the country midfield in the international ranking. This high rate of well-being is, as demonstrated, also a result of the German children's surveys.

The question that arises from an inequality theory perspective is that of what the well-being of children in these studies stands for and how the data collected by interviewing children directly about their well-being should be interpreted—overall the empirical results reveal very high scores for Germany, with only partially varying rates of agreement across various ethnic groups and social milieus/classes. This question is particularly pertinent in view of the likewise empirically established unequal opportunities of children in the family, in their leisure time activities and in school.

Confusing in Germany are the high scores in the performance context of school, for instance. As mentioned above "modern parents" expect high performance and good marks from their children (Fölling-Albers et al., 2005), teachers stipulate high performance and hard work, yet, it has been conclusively shown that especially children from lower social classes and children of Turkish origin fail to fulfil these requirements as expected, in spite of their own efforts (exemplary: Jünger, 2008).

The high satisfaction values also appear paradoxical in the family context. Children from the presumably modern, equal and symmetrical negotiation households declare both that they feel (very) good and at the same time, that

---

[10]It should be noted that in the question of "subjective well-being" UNICEF uses indicators that refer to over 11-year-olds only, and in particular to 15-year-olds (UNICEF, 2007). The age groups in German children's surveys address predominantly younger age groups than the international comparative outlook. A direct comparison of the results is thus impossible, as well-being varies with the age.

- they receive little to no pocket money from their parents and are thus financially very dependent (Betz, 2008; WVD, 2007, empirical findings on satisfied poor children with no pocket money: Chassé, Zander, & Rasch, 2003)
- only just over half (56%) of the mothers take their opinions "rather seriously" and only 47% of the fathers (WVD, 2007, p. 217)[11]
- their parents decide the outcome of the majority (86%) of conflicts between parents and children and the children, by their own accounts, must often "subordinate themselves" (Betz, 2008, p. 257ff.)
- their parents (also) resort to punishment when they are angry with the children (cf. Chapter 2).

Bearing these findings in mind, it can be assumed that the self-reported well-being of children is lower, if they regularly perceive an illegitimate misbalance of power in the family regarding the generational order and disparity. Yet overall, 85% of both girls and boys rate the liberties granted them in the family as (very) positive (WVD, 2007, p. 106f.). Ergo, there are no indications that modern children would argue against generation relations or, for instance, question their parents' authority to a greater extent than in times past, demanding an "equal footing" for negotiations.

This is but one example in support of the idea that the well-being concept should be questioned from an inequality theory perspective. After all, it conceals inequality moments in the family, as well as in other contexts that can be substantiated in modern children's lives.

In fact, the high well-being values lead to the conclusion that children honour the generational inequality conditions inherent in the generational order—just as they accept social and ethnic inequalities. They accept them as legitimate and "natural", take them as a given and (therefore) themselves participate in establishing this order and the existing conditions, just as described by Bourdieu (1976, p. 318ff.; 2005).

It is therefore vital that future children's surveys include the "well-being" variable as a self-report in order to examine children's acceptance of the existing generational order and social order and the associated balance of power. From this perspective (subjective) well-being shows the extent of the children's acceptance of existing inequality conditions, and can be viewed and interpreted as an indicator for the consent of children and their acceptance of the current inequality conditions in different areas.[12]

---

[11] In a school context, lower values were recorded: According to the children, only 26% of the teachers took their opinions "rather seriously" (girls: 30%, boys: 23%) (WVD, 2007, p. 217).

[12] In the future, internationally oriented studies should be examined more closely with regard to the interests of the researchers and policy makers involved, e.g. conceptualizing risk behaviour of young people (inter alia smoking and drunkenness) or also school aspects such as "average mean literacy scores" and "youth NEET rates" (youth not in employment, education or training) as aspects of the well-being of children and feeding the transnational findings and the league tables built thereupon into the political system.

5 Outlook: Disastrous Consequences of a Skewed Perception of Childhood

It has been empirically proven that there is little population sensitivity when the child category is assumed to be a uniform variable. In fact, the generalizing formula "modern children" and its characteristics, which are sometimes aggregated to a countrywide indicator, obscure the various albeit systematic variants of childhood and children's lives (e.g. Bühler-Niederberger & van Krieken, 2008). This neglects the synchronicity of that which is classified as non-synchronous using the terminology "traditional versus modern" (Zinnecker, 2001), as well as the different probabilities with which specific child groups can make their mark on the prevalent perceptions of modern childhood patterns, even beyond county borders.

The potential of children's surveys lies in the fact that they are a representative form of long-term monitoring of social change and the documentation of its consequences for the social group of children. The surveys can serve to empirically validate the generalizing modernization phenomena in children's lives.

Yet, this is not—as demonstrated—a sufficient basis for sensitive monitoring. Rather, a number of criteria are necessary to further develop the monitoring of childhood and (the well-being of) children. This calls for a coherent inequality theory focus and thus a sociological foundation of the related research including the direct surveying and the inequality theoretical interpretation of the well-being of children. Furthermore, it would be relevant to include all child groups, as well as the consistent monitoring of all differentiation criteria, including intersectionality of the different inequality axes.

Such a new research field and the continuous validation of modernization diagnoses would be of great relevance for a number of reasons:

First, the generalized diagnoses of changes and the homogenous perceptions of contemporary children's lives have observable consequences. Changes in the family and the lifeworld of children are seen, for instance, as sources for changes in the relationship between home and primary school, and for changes in lessons (Kirk et al., 2005). On a professional level, they lead to the postulation that children at primary school level should be dealt with differently than in the past, new media should be integrated into lessons and children should be more involved in decision making at school. On a child welfare policy level, too, markers for sound, future-oriented child welfare policy are derived from the prevalent descriptions of modern childhood patterns (MSJK, 2005, Santos Pais, 2008).

Second, this research field would also gain relevance from the fact that the prevalent perception of a homogenous child population leads to associated phenomena for those children who do not fit the perceptual mould of the modern child. For instance, one must pose the question in which way and to what extent the living situations of poor children differ from that which is considered the modern norm (Chassé et al., 2003, p. 48). Since the perceptions of and findings on modern children's lives become the norm for everyone,[13] childhood patterns that do not fit this norm become delegitimized. They are described as abnormal, traditional and thus backward—regardless of the fact that the prevalent perceptions put forward by researchers, policy makers and professionals in the field merely portray a fictive, average modern child.

References

African Child Policy Forum. (2008). *The African report on child wellbeing: How child-friendly are African governments?* Addis Ababa, Ethiopia: African Child Policy Forum.

Alanen, L. (2002). Women's studies – Childhood studies: Anknüpfungspunkte, Parallelen und Perspektiven. *Olympe – Feministische Arbeitshefte zur Politik, 16,* 46–56.

Alt, C. (2005). *Kinderleben – Aufwachsen zwischen Familie, Freunden und Institutionen* (Vol. 1). Wiesbaden, Germany: VS-Verlag.

Ben-Arieh, A. (2008). The child indicator movement: Past, present, and future. *Child Indicators Research, 1*(1), 3–16.

Bertram, H. (2006). *Zur Lage der Kinder in Deutschland. Politik für Kinder als Zukunftsgestaltung.* (Innocenti Working Paper No. 2006-2). Florence, Italy: UNICEF Innocenti Research Centre.

Bertram, H. (2008). Deutsches Mittelmaß: Der schwierige Weg in die Moderne. In H. Bertram (Ed.), *Mittelmaß für Kinder. Der UNICEF-Bericht zur Lage der Kinder in Deutschland* (pp. 37–81). Bonn, Germany: Bundeszentrale für politische Bildung.

Bertram, H., & Kohl, S. (2010). *Zur Lage der Kinder in Deutschland 2010: Kinder stärken für eine ungewisse Zukunft.* Cologne, Germany: Deutsches Komitee für UNICEF.

Betz, T. (2008). *Ungleiche Kindheiten. Theoretische und empirische Analysen zur Sozialberichterstattung über Kinder.* Weinheim, Germany: Juventa.

Betz, T. (2009). „Ich fühl' mich wohl". Zustandsbeschreibungen ungleicher Kindheiten der Gegenwart. *Diskurs Kindheits- und Jugendforschung, 4*(4), 457–470.

Bourdieu, P. (1976). *Entwurf einer Theorie der Praxis auf der ethnologischen Grundlage der kabylischen Gesellschaft.* Frankfurt am Main, Germany: Suhrkamp.

Bourdieu, P. (2005). *Die männliche Herrschaft.* Frankfurt am Main, Germany: Suhrkamp.

Bradshaw, J., Hoelscher, P., & Richardson, D. (2006). *Comparing child-well-being in OECD-countries: Concepts and methods.* Florence, Italy: UNICEF Innocent Research Centre.

Bradshaw, J., Hoelscher, P., & Richardson, D. (2007). An index of child well-being in the European union. *Social Indicators Research, 80*(1), 133–177.

Bühler-Niederberger, D. (2009). Ungleiche Kindheiten – alte und neue Disparitäten. *Aus Politik und Zeitgeschichte, 17,* 3–8.

Bühler-Niederberger, D., & van Krieken, R. (2008). Persisting inequalities: Childhood between global influences and local traditions. *Childhood, 15*(2), 147–155.

Chassé, K.-A., Zander, M., & Rasch, K. (2003). *Meine Familie ist arm. Wie Kinder im Grundschulalter Armut erleben und bewältigen.* Opladen, Germany: Leske + Budrich.

Dencik, L. (1995). Modern childhood in the Nordic countries: „dual socialisation" and its implications. In L. Chisholm (Ed.), *Growing up in Europe. Contemporary Horizons in Childhood and Youth Studies* (pp. 105–120). Berlin, Germany: Walter de Gruyter.

---

[13] Kötters (2000) writes that the modern basic pattern of parent–child relationships, inter alia respecting the child's interests, is a claim that has not found complete fulfilment in all families (ibid., p. 151). At the same time she writes that the "command household" is an obsolescent model. Such formulations give cause for investigating which groups of stakeholders formulate such claims and of what kind of norm conformance pressure this places on families and children.

du Bois-Reymond, M. (1994). Die moderne Familie als Verhandlungshaushalt. Eltern-Kind-Beziehungen in West- und Ostdeutschland und in den Niederlanden. In M. du Bois-Reymond et al. (Eds.), *Kinderleben. Modernisierung von Kindheit im interkulturellen Vergleich* (pp. 137–219). Opladen, Germany: Leske + Budrich.

du Bois-Reymond, M. (2005). Neue Lernformen – neues Generationenverhältnis? In H. Hengst & H. Zeiher (Eds.), *Kindheit soziologisch* (pp. 227–244). Wiesbaden, Germany: VS-Verlag.

Fölling-Albers, M. (2005): Soziokulturelle Bedingungen der Kindheit. In W. Einsiedler et al. (Eds.), *Handbuch Grundschulpädagogik und -didaktik* (pp. 155–166). Bad Heilbrunn, Germany: Klinkhardt.

Fuhs, B. (2002). Kindheit, Freizeit, Medien. In H. H. Krüger & C. Grunert (Eds.), *Handbuch der Kindheits- und Jugendforschung* (pp. 637–651). Opladen, Germany: Leske + Budrich.

Gille, M., Sardei-Biermann, S., Gaiser, W., & de Rijke, J. (2006). *Jugendliche und junge Erwachsene in Deutschland. Lebensverhältnisse, Werte und gesellschaftliche Beteiligung 12-bis 29-Jähriger*. Wiesbaden, Germany: VS-Verlag.

Hamburger, F., & Stauf, E. (2009). „Migrationshintergrund" zwischen Statistik und Stigma. Denkanstoß zu einem häufig verwendeten Begriff. *SCHÜLER. Wissen für Lehrer. Schüler 2009: Migration, 15*, 30–31.

Honig, M.-S. (1999). *Entwurf einer Theorie der Kindheit*. Frankfurt am Main, Germany: Suhrkamp.

James, A., & James, A. (2004). *Constructing childhood. Theory, policy and social practice.* London, England: Palgrave Macmillan.

Jünger, R. (2008). *Bildung für alle? Die schulischen Logiken von ressourcenprivilegierten und -nichtprivilegierten Kindern als Ursache der bestehenden Bildungsungleichheit.* Wiesbaden, Germany: VS-Verlag.

Kirk, S. (2005). Eltern und Schule. In W. Einsiedler et al. (Eds.), *Handbuch Grundschulpädagogik und -didaktik* (pp. 245–251). Bad Heilbrunn, Germany: Klinkhardt.

Kötters, C. (2000). *Wege aus der Kindheit in die Jugendphase*. Opladen, Germany: Leske + Budrich.

Kränzl-Nagl, R., & Mierendorff, J. (2008). Kindheit im Wandel – Annäherung an ein komplexes Phänomen. *Sozialwissenschaftliche Literatur Rundschau, 47*(1), 5–28.

LBS-Initiative Junge Familie. (2009). *LBS-Kinderbarometer Deutschland 2009. Wir sagen euch mal was. Stimmungen, Meinungen & Trends von Kindern in Deutschland.* Berlin, Germany: Bundesgeschäftsstelle der Landesbausparkassen.

Mierendorff, J. (2008). Kindheit und Wohlfahrtsstaat. In E. Luber & B. Hungerland (Eds.), *Angewandte Kindheitswissenschaften. Eine Einführung für Studium und Praxis* (pp. 199–217). Weinheim, Germany: Juventa.

Ministerium für Schule, Jugend und Kinder (MSJK). (2005). *Kinder und Jugendliche fördern – Bildung und Erziehung als Aufgabe der Kinder- und Jugendhilfe.* 8. Kinder- und Jugendbericht der Landesregierung NRW. Düsseldorf, Germany.

Noll, H.-H. (2004). Social indicators and quality of life research: Background, achievements and current trends. In N. Genov (Ed.), *Advances in sociological knowledge over half a century* (pp. 151–181). Wiesbaden, Germany: VS-Verlag.

OECD. (2009): *Doing better for children*. Paris, France: OECD Publishing.

Qvortrup, J. (2005). Kinder und Kindheit in der Sozialstruktur. In H. Hengst & H. Zeiher (Eds.), *Kindheit soziologisch* (pp. 27–47). Wiesbaden, Germany: VS-Verlag.

Roppelt, U. (2003). *Kinder – Experten ihres Alltags?* Frankfurt am Main, Germany: Peter Lang.

Santos Pais, M. (2008). Kinder als Zukunft: Warum die Lebenssituation von Kindern durch internationale Vergleiche zur Lebenslage verbessert werden kann. In H. Bertram (Ed.), *Mittelmaß für Kinder. Der UNICEF-Bericht zur Lage der Kinder in Deutschland* (pp. 220–227). Bonn, Germany: Bundeszentrale für politische Bildung.

UNICEF. (2007). *Child poverty in perspective: An overview of child well-being in rich countries.* Innocenti Report Card 7. Florence, Italy: UNICEF Innocenti Research Centre.

Wild, E. (2004). Häusliches Lernen. Forschungsdesiderate und Forschungsperspektiven. *Zeitschrift für Erziehungswissenschaft, 7*(3rd Suppl.), 37–64.

Wilk, L., & Bacher, J. (1994). *Kindliche Lebenswelten. Eine sozialwissenschaftliche Annäherung.* Opladen, Germany: Leske + Budrich.

World Vision Deutschland e. V. (WVD). (2007). *Kinder in Deutschland* 2007. 1. *World Vision Kinderstudie.* Bonn, Germany: Bundeszentrale für politische Bildung.

Zinnecker, J. (2001). Children in young and aging societies: The order of generations and models of childhood in comparative perspective. In S. L. Hofferth & T. J. Owens (Eds.), *Children at the millennium: Where have we come from, where are we going?* (pp. 11–52). Amsterdam, Netherlands: JAI Press.

Children, the Feminist Ethic of Care and Childhood Studies: Is This the Way to the Good Life?

Tom Cockburn

1 Introduction

The historian Colin Heywood (2001) in his *History of Childhood* provocatively suggests that for medieval writers, the care of children did not matter. For those in the medieval period, the natures with which we are born determine the paths of our lives and where we will end up. Such determinism was replaced with the blossoming of enlightenment thinking where notions of personhood are shaped by questions of development; the consequences of earlier life events; and the effects of child care shape how adults later experience well-being. This is perhaps the foundation to the Western approach to childhood. Indeed, care and the nature, extent and consequences of children's care are the subject of some of the most powerful modern knowledge disciplines including medicine, education, law and the social sciences. However, the disciplines have arguably been overly concerned with justifying their epistemologies and spheres of expertise over those of other competitive disciplines or 'lay' knowledge, and have created a passive image of children in requirement of treatment, education, rescue or development.

In recent years, there has been a challenge to the modernist passive child, bereft of agency, by those associated with the development of 'Childhood Studies', a loose association of anthropologists, sociologists and historians amongst others (for discussion, see Thorne, 2007). From the beginning, those associated with 'Childhood Studies' (CS) worked with an approach that would see children as social actors in their own right; who have knowledge, rights, responsibilities and understandings of the way they feel and experience their own well-being, the education they receive, the medical decisions they may make about themselves. What is quite remarkable is to see the approach of CS moving from being marginal to an almost orthodoxy within our social science disciplines.

Where CS has focused analysis on a 'newly discovered' active, agentic child, the approach that has challenged the nature and extent of care has come from feminism

T. Cockburn (✉)
Department of Social Studies and Humanities, University of Bradford, Bradford BD7 1DP, UK
e-mail: t.d.cockburn@bradford.ac.uk

S. Andresen et al. (eds.), *Children and the Good Life*, Children's Well-Being: Indicators and Research 4, DOI 10.1007/978-90-481-9219-9_3,

(although mention must also be made of those receiving care, such as service users, disabled people and, of course, children themselves). Feminists have challenged the way caring has been understood in modernity as something done to passive bodies, viewing it as a complex process where caring is done by people, on people, in contexts that are imbued with power relations. Caring, it was found, can actually be bad for you and disempowering. Care is certainly received unequally and performed by people unequally. Furthermore, feminists have challenged the 'moral reasoning' of existing knowledge that focuses on rules, laws, procedures, abstractions and facts, proposing one based around relationships and responsibilities.

This paper discusses and argues for the importance of a juxtaposition and an alliance between CS and a 'feminist ethic of care' (FEC). It does so by briefly outlining the two approaches and then offering some scenarios in which such a fusion may take place along with some ways forward.

2 Feminist Ethic of Care

The first 'wave' of the FEC begins with the publication of Carol Gilligan's *In a Different Voice*, influential in moral theory, feminism and feminist theory in general. In the book, Gilligan engaged a critique of the previous conventional moral theory associated with the developmental psychology of Lawrence Kohlberg. By way of contrast to Kohlberg's assumptions of child development where reasoning 'develops' at specific 'stages', Gilligan (1982) drew on Nancy Chodorow's (1978) gendered object relations theory to arrive at the sense where girls adopted a different set of moral reasoning to boys. According to Chodorow, mothers experience their daughters as less separate from themselves, and girls thereby are not (unlike boys) pushed away from their mothers and thereby compelled to repress their intimacy, tenderness and capacity for care. Drawing on this, Gilligan argues that girls develop a capacity for empathy and sensitivity, whereas boys define themselves in terms of independence and autonomy. According to Gilligan, 'masculine' moral reasoning utilises mathematical calculations and the adoption of hierarchical rules; by way of contrast, girls look to more concrete, relational issues to adjudicate moral dilemmas. The parallels to early sociological studies of childhood are quite marked. Childhood Studies critiqued developmental psychology as devaluing the reasoning of children in a similar way to how a woman's reasoning was marginalised. The moral reasoning that values hierarchies of expert knowledge, the rewarding of an accumulation of mathematical and technical knowledge would always place children as 'other'.

However, there were difficulties with Gilligan's early approach to the FEC. There are the much-vaunted (from the developmental psychology 'establishment') methodological weaknesses to Gilligan's work as her sampling was selective and small (Sommers, 2001). We can add that Gilligan's deployment of 'women's moral reasoning' does not deconstruct the category 'woman' and the assumption of moral superiority (see Riley, 1988). For instance, Stack's work found that there were fewer differences between the caring done on white people by African American men and woman, than those between white men and women. Furthermore, within sociology, there was a shift away from associating care with oppression and exploitation to viewing care through the framework of social obligations and normative structures where caring activities are analysed in a more nuanced way (Finch, 1989). Feminist ethicists have highlighted women's special role in caring relationships; for instance, Noddings (1984, p. 2) describes care as 'essentially feminine'. However, this unhelpfully marginalises the role of men as carers and the increasingly recognised caring done by children. For instance, 50% of the 23% of children under 16 in the UK who care for an adult, do so for more than 11 h per week (Dearden & Becker, 2004, p. 5). Statistics so far collected in the UK are measurements of children caring for adults only and do not count the largest proportion of caring by children that is directed at their siblings, for which there are no reliable figures. As Brannen and Heptinstall (2003, p. 195) argue, "children emerge as active co-participants in care and constructors of family life". Although we can assume that this is also gendered, as girls are drawn into this caring role more than boys, it is not exclusively so. Indeed, most feminist writers now avoid such essentialist thinking and instead focus on the processes whereby activities of caring (mostly performed by women but also by others) are marginalised in today's society.

Nevertheless, Gilligan's work was hugely influential and was built upon by other moral theorists such as Joan Tronto (1993) who developed the ethic of care to include a total world view which includes

> Everything we do to maintain, continue and repair our 'world' so that we can live in it as well as possible. That world includes our bodies, our selves and our environment, all of which we seek to interweave in a complex, life-sustaining web (p. 103).

In this 'second wave' of the FEC, definitions of care are placed within broader social and political concerns rather than essentialised individual-gendered psychology. For Tronto, care is a more complicated phenomenon, and an ethic of care takes the position of the others' needs into account. Tronto develops four ethical elements of care including attentiveness to the process of caring about someone; responsibility to those that we take care of; levels of competence involved in giving care; and responsiveness of those receiving care. A full account of Tronto's treatise is beyond the word limits of this chapter, but the important point is the awareness she shows of the power differentials where caring about and taking care of people are often the duties of the powerful. By way of contrast, the concrete giving and receiving of care are left to the least powerful in society.

In terms of a moral theory and how the good life is to be achieved, Tronto identifies three 'moral boundaries' that are helpful to reflect upon. First, traditional moral theory separates public and private life. Those such as children are cared for in 'private' spaces and are absent, excluded or 'protected' from public life. While issues of privacy are of course fundamental to our good life, feminists over the past century have shown that private spaces are often sites of loneliness, violence and abuse experienced by women and children. The challenge to the public/private distinction leads to the second 'moral boundary' which challenges the separation of morality from politics. Politicians have long been subjected to scandals. However, arguably deeper moral questions such as the nature of education, the feelings of the sick and social questions beyond economic and political efficiency are just as valid. Due to feminist and other challenges to political life, moral issues such as corporal punishment have entered the political realm and led to important reforms. The final 'moral boundary' concerns challenges to abstract accounts of morality and builds upon Gilligan's critique of technical and expert-led solutions to questions of the 'good life' and instead to challenges to top-down definitions of well-being. This is an important point where measurements of well-being are placed within quantitative frameworks that are separated from the lifeworlds of children. Interestingly, the quantitative methods in this collection have developed their indicators and measurements in conversations with and references to CS.

The new moral theory associated with the FEC offers a new way of thinking about politics and society. However, recent usages of the FEC have developed what I will call a 'third wave' that has applied the philosophy to particular contexts in the real world but, at the same time, utilises the benefits of technical approaches embedded in realist and positivistic epistemologies. By doing so, two fundamental caveats must be applied: first, as Sevenhuijsen (1998) has argued, the FEC must not be conflated with what she called the 'mothering paradigm' that is associated only with women and fails to recognise the sometimes oppressive nature of caring; second, as I have argued elsewhere (Cockburn, 2005, 2007), ethics of care and developments of traditional moral theory must not be placed as polar opposites. Instead, principles according to justice, economics, materialism and 'science' do have important contributions to make in furthering children's well-being. Kröger (2009) has the same thing in mind when arguing that the relationships between disabled people and their care assistants share the care relationship and require a balancing of the needs and interests of the two parties. Conversely, access to adequate care could be perceived as a human right. What is of overwhelming importance is to place all of these moral theories into some sense of dialogue. Sevenhuijsen (1998, 2004), for instance, correctly advocates placing ethical and moral debates within the context of pluralism and democratic citizenship; where technical, 'expert-led' forms of knowledge are questioned, challenged and debated rather than merely accepted.

In my view, the FEC offers a vital added value to other moral approaches, as the approach demands that hypothetical and policy dilemmas cannot be divorced from the immediate realities and emotional complexities of people's lives. Cogently, Porter (1999, p. 5) describes the example where "if you are surrounded by the demands of small children, the confusion of teenagers or the needs of ageing relatives, then the considerations needed to make moral choices differ from those who only need to consider themselves".

Thus, it is central to understand the processes of caring by focusing on actual, concrete and connected settings. For instance, in child welfare policy, the principle of 'protecting children from harm' must be applied to the specific context of a confused or vulnerable child that can be lost amidst policy and legal 'procedures'. The ethic of care highlights principles of equity and inclusion and sees 'emotional detachment' as irrelevant or even an anathema to good quality caring. The connected nature of caring must be aware of the 'moral deliberation' associated with care (Sevenhuijsen, 1998, p. 128). Caring involves differential elements of responsibilities and need and often includes conflicting agendas. Thus, a caring ethical framework must be deliberative and involve situated social practices that are "open-textured, dialogic, open to criticism, self-criticism and debate" (ibid.). Here it is not just top-down knowledge that requires watching but also knowledge within the concrete contexts of caring for and being cared for.

3 Children and Well-Being

John O'Neill (2000) has identified four structures where children are exposed to social, economic, psychological and biological risks:

   (i) child exposure to biorisks in the uterine environment;
  (ii) child exposure to biopsychic and sociopsychological risks in the domestic environment;
 (iii) child exposure to socioeconomic risks on the class environment of the family;
 (iv) child exposure to global environmental risks in the family and community (p. 89).

From this breakdown, we can discern clear links in the well-being of children to that of their mothers, families and communities. All of these risks are compounded by social class and poverty. O'Neill's responses to these risks are not to bolster ideologies of familism, privacy and feminising childcare, paternal delinquency or welfare dependency. Instead, rather similar to Sevenhuijsen's (1998) ideas around the FEC, he argues for a 'civic' notion of civil society where children's well-being is based on the following assumptions: children's well-being is secured through more complex and intensive interactions with primary caretakers; children's development is improved where the home interacts and overlaps with the broader social and civic environment; the child, parents, siblings, school and neighbourhood are congruent and in communication with each other and balance their competing demands upon the child. This reflects interest in developing an 'ecological' approach to child welfare that places interactions of the child, family, schools, community and society as central to any analysis (Bronfenbrenner, 1979).

Today's approach to children's well-being can be characterised into what Isaiah Berlin (1958) called 'negative liberty'; that is, the idea of rights and freedoms that identify parameters to the acts of individuals pursuing their own interests. The application to our contemporary societies is the characteristic where one is compelled to 'tolerate', or not disturb the projects of others. These include requirements where someone is not permitted to engage in or abstains from certain actions. Here, one can think of many situations of children and their carers, such as the requirement *not* to physically injure children in their care. The problem that arises, Udovicki notes, is that it does not provide any recommendations on what people should do instead, given any particular situation. These duties of omission are not sufficient 'to sustain a relationship of fellowship and love' (Udovicki, 1993, p. 53). In this case, merely preventing injuries to children, Udovicki argues, does not 'reach far enough psychologically to motivate a "fellow feeling". . . [and] does not encourage actively helping others to obtain their relevant objectives and desires' (ibid.). Thus, preventing the physical punishment of children does not foster the dissemination of alternative ways of guiding children. Additionally, these acts of 'tolerance' being applied universally fail to promote other virtues, such as viewing the perspective of others, friendship and the reciprocity of love.

Within social policy, care is placed within the discourses of individualism and inserted into frameworks around 'rights' and 'responsibilities'. As Sevenhuijsen (2000) has noted in her analysis of the 'Third Way', an approach so deeply influential in the UK New Labour programme, the operation of 'rights' assumes a choice about what we do and the corresponding duties or responsibilities, such as those around care. Yet this 'usually offers little space for reflection about how people actually experience or "do" responsibilities, or for the moral considerations they employ in that respect' (Sevenhuijsen, 2004, p. 28). The 'Third Way' persists in the assumption that people are primarily calculating, rational beings who weigh economic benefits and costs to their actions. While economic calculations are, of course, important in people's deliberations, they are not the only consideration. Those who offer care have a variety of motives beyond the economic. Furthermore, reducing care to a 'cost' or 'duty' places those in dependency in a devalued position.

Welcome though welfare initiatives are, these initiatives are still centred more around technical delivery of services than reformulating caring ethics. As Brannen and Moss (2003, p. 207), who advocate an ethic of care, have warned us, 'current instrumental approaches— technical, managerial, normalizing and universalistic— which are underpinned by market or business ethics, an "ethic of care" approach would seek ways to work with diversity, complexity and uncertainty'.

Care remains a distinct policy that is separated artificially from education, health and criminal justice. Instead, care should, as Brannen and Moss (2003, p. 199) have argued, 'become a way of acting and a habit of mind informing education, health and other domains—a manifestation of a "caring" society applied across all public services and other human services agencies'.

Commentators who seek to include children in citizenship have emphasised the ways governments should move away from a closed controlling and steering government towards one that is open to a conversation and dialogue with children (Roche, 1999). Those advocating FEC have similarly identified a public sphere that needs to 'become acquainted with the stories of others. . . they will arrive at "shared meanings"' (Sevenhuijsen 2003, p. 15). There is reason for optimism in seeking to encourage this more dialogical governance, in that wider social changes around care are taking place in society. This is possibly due to the movement of women into public organisations where they can introduce caring into these spaces. First, 'caring professions', such as health, are moving from mere 'acute' services to palliative and preventative services that allow the nature and type of care to be taken seriously. Relatedly, 'user groups' are increasingly being brought into the planning and delivery of services; children are a large and important 'user group' whose views are beginning to be sought. Second, men are also increasing their caring in both formal and informal settings. While there is still a good deal of ground to make up, the mould has been broken and the traditional taboos of men carers are weakening. Finally, caring is moving out of the private sphere and is now located across the public, voluntary and private sectors. Caring is big business. While this has huge disadvantages, it does signify a movement in how caring is beginning to be taken seriously. Debates around caring and the inclusion of ethical deliberations have never been as timely (Sevenhuijsen & Svab, 2003). As Sevenhuijsen and Svab (2003, pp. 37–38) have argued, the location of care to the public sphere 'confronts us with the necessity and possibility of using the moral orientation of care in our public agency: acting together with a view to creating a sustainable and dignified existence for everyone'.

4 Feminism and Childhood Studies

This section draws on the important work of Berry Mayall (2003) who has explored the tensions between feminism and the burgeoning CS literature that she correctly describes as a social movement as well as an intellectual approach. One key aspect has been the focus that feminists tend to apply to children are mainly around issues of childcare and child abuse. For feminists, the key focus is on women's involvement in childcare and men as abusers, and children are, on the whole, presented as languidly receiving care and as passive victims of abuse, mostly by men. For feminists, attention has centred on childcare and daycare issues. There has also been feminist attention to children in the socialisation process, where boys and girls acquire their gender role expectations. Again, as Mayall has pointed out, children are presented as passive to this process.

The lessons learned from the recent work of sociologists associated with CS should, nevertheless, find close alliance with feminism. The conflict in interests between women and children only applies to the fact that mothers are pressured to be paid workers and carry the *single* responsibility for childcare. Here children are not the 'question' for women, but the contemporary labour market, men's participation in caring and the operation of the welfare state. Thus, feminism and CS can be symbiotic allies in creating a better world for women, children and men.

First, children's vulnerability is socially constructed through masculine-ordered social environments. For children, the fact that women are moving into these environments and taking up positions of power means that these environments can change and be constructed to allow children's own agency to be recognised. For instance, Mayall uses the example of Finland, where mothers work in partnership with the state to facilitate children to live competent and independent lives. This has the consequence of children and mothers living more independently, and the state has the benefit of developing competent and empowered young citizens.

Second, having feminists who recognise that children are active and not passive in households allows for a more accurate understanding of how children, parents, neighbourhoods and institutions interact. The work of Suzanne Hood (1999) has shown how children are central to negotiations between the school and the home.

By beginning to understand children as competent social actors, it can be seen that children act as the definers of how the school interacts with parents and how the school understands the home through the child. Children therefore are important ambassadors of the family and community; engaging with these children in the fullest sense promotes the interests of all the stakeholders.

Third, taking children seriously as competent social actors allows for an exact understanding of caring within private and public relationships. An understanding of how caring happens allows for children's and women's 'hidden work' to be recognised, and it can facilitate a mutually fulfilling dialogue. This can only benefit women, children and men too, as 'vulnerabilities' and 'dependency' are reformulated in ways that may allow greater and more fulfilling relationships for all.

5 Formation of Alliances

The well-being of children requires help and assistance from adults. Needless to say this assistance usually comes not only from family and friends but also from communities—as characterised by the now famous maxim that it takes a village to raise a child. Family and cultural life are mediated through a wide spectrum of cultures in specific contexts. Much of the burgeoning literature around CS focuses on this context of children's relationships with communities, peers and families and has placed children's voices not as passive recipients of culture and families but as active participants and co-creators of family and community life. Throughout Northern societies, family life has been transformed through the sexual revolution and the pluralisation of family forms (Jensen, 2009). Or, as many feminists have observed, the boundaries between the public and private have changed as more women/mothers go out for paid employment outside the home (Lohan, 2000).

The movement of mothers and the number of women spending time in the public sphere has led to changes in the nature of the public sphere. In many respects, it becomes more amenable to diversities, and previously held private issues have become public. This includes issues concerning children; children's lives are becoming more 'institutionalised' as they spend more time in paid care from a young age and long hours in schools and at after-school facilities (Zeiher, 2009). In fact, the 'children's workforce' in the UK forms a significant proportion of the workforce as carers, play workers, nurses and educators. One recent estimate in the UK places the figure at over 2.7 million, with a further six million volunteers (Children's Workforce Network, 2009, p. 4). There are clearly shared interests with the children in their care, as the sector has high levels of low-paid, part-time and casual contracts. It is important that those working with children be respected by appropriate pay and conditions, as this will lead arguably to better quality care of children.

Relatedly, the state's role in the caring of children has accelerated, especially in the last 30 years, and there has been a 'professionalisation' of practitioners in the children's workforce—be they social workers, nurses or teachers. Writers, such as Parton (2002), have highlighted the ways in which the state has drifted towards elements of surveillance and control, often undermining the trust placed with parents, especially in poor households. Feminists have focused on issues of 'over-exhaustion' of professionals, and the decline in status of caregivers and the FEC has been applied to professional contexts, highlighting the need for attentiveness and responsiveness to those in their care (Lloyd, 2005). This is in marked contrast to 'masculinist' and 'bureaucratic' solutions to care. Thus, the importance of context of caring and professionalisation becomes important; this attention to context is something the writers associated with CS have nearly always emphasised in their conclusions. Furthermore, there is a long tradition of a 'radical' perspective in social care in general, as writers since Donald Schön (1983) accentuate the importance of social contexts and 'swampy ground' of practice that remains a sharp distinction to the more bureaucratic 'outcomes-led' approaches of recent times. Recently, there has been a development of 'service-user' movements around disability, mental health and some children and young people that advocate and campaign for those who are 'cared for'; they provide a platform or a voice, guard against the dangers of professional power, and attend to the disempowering condition and 'infantilisation' associated with 'over-caring'.

Most professionals in the child welfare field are firmly committed to principles of empowerment of children and their families. Empowerment is not to be addressed through the deliverance of 'gifts' of welfare, but through the encouragement of collective self-help that can only be achieved through encouraging people with similar socially structured problems to share experiences and appreciate the shared nature of their problems (Wise, 1995). In terms of the 'listening to children' agenda, the voices of children must not be individualised but rather placed alongside those of other children with shared interests. This is being done in the UK to some extent with groups of children, such as those in the 'looked after' sector and those children with disabilities (although this is far from universal practice). However, for most disadvantaged children, having professionals who encourage a shared consciousness is placed very low on the agenda, if it is there at all. The FEC, if utilised, moves care away from the politics of employment and social services to care as a form of social participation and democratic practice.

The contemporary circumstances of family life, community contexts, increasing professional and state power allows an important role for CS. CS originates from the long social scientific tradition of obtaining and theorising empirical data. The approach of the social sciences has accumulated over 100 years' experience in focusing on social practices and seeks to understand interpretative traditions, including those around care. Importantly, as noted above, the disciplines have largely moved away from crude psychologism and rationalism to an epistemology interested in culture and meanings that recognises human agency and interdependence. CS has applied these tools to children and now sees children as active constructors of their social worlds. CS scholars, by challenging children's passivity in the face of psychological, medical and other care discourses, does not need too much of a radical break to politicise processes of care, as feminists have done in recent times. We should not be limited to the interpretative tradition, as many of the articles in this collection have utilised the radical epistemology of CS to develop quantitative tools, variables and indicators to measure, compare and chart children's well-being in a variety of countries across the globe. Any ethic of care for and by children needs to be informed by such data.

The newly emerging 'third wave' of the FEC and CS complement each other. Both approaches are keenly aware of very similar issues, such as the importance of diversity and the subtle nature of discrimination and disempowerment. Both approaches are also aware of the subtle resistances of marginalised people, and both theorise how voices and personhood become devalued and irrationalised. They also share a requirement for a radical critique of social policy and political practices. Rather similar to how all men have benefited from women as empowered, interesting and more independent companions and friends, so too would men and women benefit from empowered, interesting and more independent children. Being with, caring for and being cared by after all is an essential precondition of the good life for all of us.

References

Berlin, I. (1958). *Two concepts of liberty*. Oxford, England: Clarendon Press.

Brannen, J., & Heptinstall, E. (2003). Concepts of care and children's contribution to family life. In J. Brannen & P. Moss (Eds.), *Rethinking children's care* (pp. 183–197). Buckingham, England: Open University Press.

Brannen, J., & Moss, P. (2003). Some thoughts on rethinking children's care. In J. Brannen & P. Moss (Eds.), *Rethinking children's care* (pp. 198–209). Buckingham, England: Open University Press.

Bronfenbrenner, U. (1979). *The ecology of human development: Experiments by nature and design*. Cambridge, MA: Harvard University Press.

Children's Workforce Network. (2009). *Researching common issues that affect mobility within the children and young peoples' workforce*. www.childrensworkforce.org.uk/.../Research_into _Common_Issues_Affecting_Mobility_Across_the_Children_s_Workforce.pdf. Accessed October 2009.

Chodorow, N. (1978). *The reproduction of mothering*. Berkeley, CA: University of California Press.

Cockburn, T. (2005). Children and the feminist ethic of care. *Childhood: A Global Journal of Child Research, 12*(1), 71–89.

Cockburn, T. (2007). Reconstructing children's agency: Boundaries of 'rights' and 'care'. In C. Beckett, O. Heathcote, & M. Macey (Eds.), *Negotiating boundaries: Identities, sexualities, diversities* (pp. 155–166). Newcastle, England: Cambridge Scholars Press.

Dearden, C., & Becker, S. (2004). *Young carers in the UK*. London, England: The Children's Society.

Finch, J. (1989). *Family obligations and social change*. Cambridge, England: Polity.

Gilligan, C. (1982). *In a different voice*. Boston: Harvard University Press.

Heywood, C. (2001). *History of childhood*. Cambridge, England: Polity.

Hood, S. (1999). Home-school agreements: A true partnership. *School Leadership and Management, 21*(1), 7–17.

Jensen, A.-M. (2009). Pluralization of family forms. In J. Qvortrup, A. Corsaro, & M.-S. Honig (Eds.), *The Palgrave handbook of children's studies* (pp. 140–155). Basingstoke, England: Palgrave Macmillan.

Kröger, T. (2009). Care research and disability studies: Nothing in common? *Critical Social Policy, 29*, 398–414.

Lloyd, L. (2005). A caring profession? *British Journal of Social Work, 36*(7), 1171–1185.

Lohan, M. (2000). Come back public/private. *Women's Studies International Forum, 23*(1), 107–117.

Mayall, B. (2003). Generation and gender: Childhood studies and feminism. In B. Mayall (Ed.), *Childhood in generational perspective* (pp. 87–110). London, England: Social Science Research Unit, Institute of Education, University of London.

Noddings, N. (1984). *Caring: A feminine approach to ethics and moral education.* Berkeley, CA: University of California Press.

O'Neill, J. (2000). Cultural capitalism and child formation. In H. Cavanna (Ed.), *The new citizenship of the family: Comparative perspectives* (pp. 79–98). Aldershot, England: Ashgate.

Parton, N. (2002). Rethinking *professional* practice: The contributions of social constructionism and the feminist 'ethics of care'. *British Journal of Social Work, 33*, 1–16.

Porter, E. (1999). *Feminist perspectives on ethics.* London, England: Longman.

Riley, D. (1988). *Am I that name?* Oxford, England: Macmillan.

Roche, J. (1999). Children: Rights, participation and citizenship. *Childhood, 6*(4), 475–495.

Schön, D. (1983). *The reflective practitioner: How professionals think in action.* New York: Basic Books.

Sevenhuijsen, S. (1998). *Citizenship and the ethics of care.* London, England: Routledge.

Sevenhuijsen, S. (2000). Caring in the third way. *Critical Social Policy, 20*(1): 5–37.

Sevenhuijsen, S. (2003). The Place of Care. The Relevance of the. Ethic of Care for Social Policy. In S. Sevenhuijsen, S., & A. Svab, A. (Eds.), *Labyrinths of care* (pp. 13–41),. Ljubljana, Slovenia: Mirovni Institut

Sevenhuijsen, S. (2004). Trace: A method for normative policy analysis from the ethic of care. In S. Sevenhuijsen & A. Svab (Eds.), *The heart of the matter* (pp. 13–46). Ljubljana, Slovenia: Mirovni Institut.

Sevenhuijsen, S., & Svab, A. (2003). *Labyrinths of care.* Ljubljana, Slovenia: Mirovni Institut.

Sommers, C. (2001). *The war against boys.* New York: Touchstone Books.

Thorne, B. (2007). Authorial: Crafting the interdisciplinary field of childhood studies. *Childhood, 14*, 147–152.

Tronto, J. (1993). *Moral boundaries.* London, England: Routledge.

Udovicki, J. (1993). Justice and care in close relationships. *Hypatia, 8*(3), 48–60.

Wise, S. (1995). Feminist ethics in practice. In R. Hugman & D. Smith (Eds.), *Ethical issues in social work* (pp. 104–119). London, England: Routledge.

Zeiher, H. (2009). Institutionalization as a secular trend. In J. Qvortrup, A. Corsaro, & M.-S. Honig (Eds.), *The Palgrave handbook of childhood studies* (pp. 127–139). Basingstoke, England: Palgrave Macmillan.

Childhood Welfare and the Rights of Children

Lourdes Gaitán Muñoz

1 Introduction

This chapter is about social rights as children's rights, recognized as such in the United Nations Convention on the Rights of the Child (CRC). Understanding the CRC as a component of human rights as a whole, it is important to highlight the specific dimensions that social rights have when applied to improve children's well-being. It is well known that the CRC represents an important advance on previous international advocacy instruments on children's rights such as the Declaration on the Rights of the Child (1959)—especially regarding participation rights. But the so-named *provision* rights have gained space in the CRC too, and through explanation of the contents of these rights, the commitments of the national states and the responsibilities of parents.

This chapter starts with a general overview of human rights as citizenship rights, followed immediately by an analysis of the dimensions of provision rights for children. Some results will be reported based on our own research asking children directly about their feelings and opinions on welfare in general and their expected well-being in particular. The chapter concludes with recommendations for both policies and the adult society.

2 Social Welfare and Human Rights

Social welfare can be explained in a lot of ways. Here, we are invited to think about it in terms of values. In these terms, social welfare would be a social value assuming a collective aim to reach a fair distribution of existing social resources in order to satisfy human demands commonly accepted as needs. The human rights activist Susan George's statement on the European model of social welfare can be understood in

L.G. Muñoz (✉)
Faculty of Political Science and Sociology, Complutense University of Madrid,
Ciudad Universitaria, 28040 Madrid, Spain
e-mail: mlourdes.gaitan@wanadoo.es

S. Andresen et al. (eds.), *Children and the Good Life*, Children's Well-Being: Indicators and Research 4, DOI 10.1007/978-90-481-9219-9_4,
© Springer Science+Business Media B.V. 2010

this sense: "It is one of the greatest creations of the human spirit and we should be able to generalize it to the entire world" (El País Semanal, August 8, 2004). One might ask why this model should deserve such resounding praise, precisely at a time when this model is exposed to such strong criticism.

The idea of social welfare can be considered as a latent part of the United Nations Universal Declaration of Human Rights in 1948, when it refers to the social rights that, together with civil and political rights, make up the rights of citizenship under Marshall's (1950) well-known and extended vision. Despite the time elapsed since this declaration, both the notion of universal human rights and that of citizenship can be debated, revised and updated, but they remain higher-order aspirations for humankind.

Marshall proposes dividing citizenship into three parts dictated by history even more clearly than by logic:

1. *The civil element* is composed of the rights necessary for the individual freedom or liberty of the person; freedom of speech, thought and faith; the right to own property and to conclude valid contracts; and the right to justice.
2. *The political element* is the right to participate in the exercise of political power as a member of a body invested with political authority or as an elector of the members of such a body.
3. *The social element* covers the whole range from the right to a modicum of economic welfare and security to the right to fully share the social heritage and to live the life of a civilized being according to the standards prevailing in society. The institutions most closely connected with this are the educational system and the social services.

Marshall considered that without too much violence to historical accuracy, it is possible to assign the formative period in the life of each element to a different century: civil rights to the eighteenth, political rights to the nineteenth, and social rights to the twentieth centuries. At present, the three elements are included in the Universal Declaration of Human Rights (1948).

It is worth comparing the type of rights recognized for children with those recognized for adults in general. Looking at the childhood cycle, the first legislation was enacted in the labour area, the types of rights referring to the person did not become consolidated until the Convention and the ones having to do with their participation in social life are only emerging. Therefore, it could be said that there is an inversion in the historic order of their rights: first the social ones, then the civil ones, with the political ones still pending. However, apart from the former defensive legislation related to child labour, the social benefits for children appeared later, sketched in the 1959 Declaration and more clearly developed in the 1989 Convention.

Because of the timing of the appearance of citizenship rights, nowadays, it is common to talk about three generations of human rights: the first composed of civil and political rights; the second, social rights. The third wave of rights emerged after the Universal Declaration of Human Rights, even though based on it. These rights can be classified in two groups: those defined either by the *object* (environmental rights) or by the *subject* (women's rights, children's rights, rights of people with disabilities, etc.). Since children's rights are included in the second type, it can be said that children's rights are part of the human rights established universally as a whole.

3 The Social Welfare of Childhood

3.1 Children's Rights

The CRC is supported by social values. The well-known phrase *in the child's best interest* reflects precisely such a kind of value. But the problem is who defines best interest. There is always an adult who interprets this, translating the former values of the CRC, some kind of European-bourgeois adult values, to the present. The introduction of the Convention recalls how the Universal Declaration of Human Rights in 1948 declared that every human being has all the rights and liberties stated, and, likewise, that childhood has the right to care and special support. The Convention's focus is mainly to specify this special attention, which has a double meaning: On the one side, it reflects the national states' interest in childhood, which is translated, mainly, in terms of protection; on the other side, it represents the segregation of these small human beings into specific spaces, especially in terms of their participation and personal autonomy.

The rights recognized in the Convention were classified into the three types— Provision, Protection and Participation (the three Ps), in order to make circulation easier:

1. *Provision* refers to the right to own, receive or have access to certain resources and services; the distribution of these resources between the child and adult population.
2. *Protection* has to do with the right to receive parental and professional care and live without being subjected to abusive acts and practices.
3. *Participation* expresses the right to do things, express oneself, and have an individual and collective voice (Heiliö, Lauronen, & Bardy, 1993, p. 12).

The group of rights addressing the participation of children in society, the rights to be heard, especially on topics that affect them, is the newest one, but, at the same time, the most limited and the least developed in practice. Included under this heading are the articles referring to the right to freedom of expression, thought and conscience (with the parent's guidance); to be listened to regarding all legal or administrative procedures affecting him or her (without being able to demand judicial or administrative rights independently from parents or representatives); to liberty of association and to hold peaceful meetings (even though no mention is given to developing political activities, electing representatives or being elected). Work is also a way of participating in social life. However, this is not recognized for children from the standpoint of liberty, but from the standpoint of protection.

Protection takes up the most extensive part of the CRC, and these are the rights pertaining to the situations that are the greatest threats to children's lives. The protection agreed by all the states Parties to the Convention addresses the violation of minors' rights by parents, the family and others responsible for their well-being, as well as by institutions or persons not related to the family, such as centres or alternative living establishments set up by the national state, by the mass media or by adults trying to abuse, sell or exploit children.

The provision addressing the possibility of having access to and enjoying adequate and sufficient material resources is the aspect of the Convention related more directly to the subject of the well-being of children. Its main content is found in Articles 24–30. In Articles 24 and 25, the States Parties recognize the right of the child to enjoy the highest possible level of health and to receive periodic health examinations for any treatment she or he is undergoing. Article 26 talks about the right to benefit from social security (according to the national legislation). In Article 28, the States recognize children's right to education, and Article 29 establishes the general guidelines that education has to meet. Before this, Article 27 talks about the right of every child to an adequate standard of living to ensure physical, mental, spiritual, moral and social development, adding the following: It is the responsibility of the parents or other persons in charge of the child to provide the necessary life conditions for her or his development even though (the following paragraph from the article explains) the States will adopt proper measures to help parents be effective in complying with this right. In essence, this set of articles specifies the distribution of responsibilities in the provision of means to make welfare easier for minors. This is discussed in the following section.

Before continuing, the aspects of the Convention that stand out as the most positive ones for children's lives will be commented on, as well as the ones considered to be defects that must be overcome.

The most outstanding virtue of the Convention lies in the sole and repeated attribution of children's rights in itself, and to the fact that children are treated as individuals. Next to this it is worth mentioning that the States Parties of the Convention are the ones that recognize these rights and accept responsibility for their fulfilment, with the Convention establishing a continuous system to follow up advances achieved in the different countries in relation to the protection of these rights and the advancement of the welfare of children. Last of all, if the Convention is unable, per se, to resolve the problems affecting the individuals since they are under a certain age, it does have the capacity to make these problems more visible, establishing the foundations and adequate mechanisms to approach their resolution.

Concerning its shortcomings, the most outstanding ones are the adult-centred conception and the vision based on the dominant western culture, both latent in the text of the CRC. Let us examine the translation of each one of these aspects separately.

On the one hand, the Convention expresses a desired generational order, and this grants children access to resources according to what has been established. The protection rights, which do not touch the relations of power between adults and children, are the most developed ones, whereas the genuine participation rights that would challenge the power hierarchy between generations, are poorly developed (Agathonos, 1993). The vision of children as dependent beings and of childhood as a preparation stage is reflected upon and reinforced in the Convention. This leads to contradictions that challenge the main innovation stimulus proposed by it. For example, the second article, formulated to avoid any type of discrimination "between children", says nothing about discrimination in terms of adult rights. On the other hand, all the text refers to the individual child (even though it is important to point out that there are no references to specific problems based on the gender issue, whereas a whole article is dedicated to detail, positively, the specific guarantees to assure that the mentally or physically disabled child enjoys a complete, decent and honourable life), assuming the developmental perspective through the multiple references to maturity and the child's competence as an argument to limit capacity to act, mainly in the public arena, reducing in this manner the recognition of civil rights. Maybe what is most important in this sphere is the asymmetric relation to adults consolidated by the Convention: children are subjects with rights, but not with a responsibility to perform duties. This excludes them from the exchange relationships regulated for adults at the normative level (Gaitán, 2006).

Regarding the cultural aspect, and despite the specific reference to children belonging to ethnic, religious, linguistic or indigenous minorities (Article 30), the paradigms and categories of the dominant western development model prevail in the Convention's text. As Recknagel (2002, p. 19) points out, "Mono-cultural and ethnocentric concepts about the rights obstruct any focus on the particularities of the cultures and communities" (translated). Without falling into a perspective of cultural relativism, and thereby justifying unacceptable behaviours towards children, this author examines three aspects of the Convention (child labour, health and education). Recknagel analyses the CRC from a cultural difference perspective, and highlights the possible need for a reformulation of the text. His recommendations can be summarized as follows: Regarding child labour, a different point of view should be maintained (protection against exploitation instead of prohibiting child labour) highlighting the positive role of labour in children's socialization, not only for indigenous or rural communities but also for children in western societies. In relation to health, he proposes that, alongside the main health service based on western principles of official medicine, local nutrition practices and the structures of traditional health should be promoted and recognized. Regarding education, the author finds it necessary to include the appraisal of the oral tradition and local knowledge, not in order to replace the current article, but rather as a complement to modern western educational contents.

3.2 The Deal Between Society, the Family and the State

The family orientation is present throughout the entire text of the CRC. It proves to be quite explicit in respect to the rights and duties of parents, and in a certain way, it permeates considerations on the responsibilities of the states and the societies. Once again, this reflects the dominant thought characterized by the tendency to consider that children belong to their parents "by nature". Their physical framework is the home, and the family is the medium in which their primary relations develop. This also marks the path for the secondary relations, social status, values and ways of behaving the child will end up adopting. In this way, the child's social identity is like a mirror of her or his parents' life, and, at the same time, the family is portrayed by the type of child it produces. Because of this, when the child is an object of criticism, the parents are to blame (Makrinioti, 1994; Qvortrup, 1990). This does not mean that the governments can evade any responsibility in relation to children. On the contrary, with prevention as a target, they have indirect responsibilities to promote and maintain the abilities and capacities of the parents and, in a subsidiary way, direct responsibilities over the child's welfare if the parents do not tend to their duties properly.

Article 27 of the Convention mentioned above shows an example of how the interplay of these responsibilities is produced. The article indicates, in its second section, that "the parent(s) or others responsible for the child have the primary responsibility to secure *within their abilities and financial capacities*, the conditions of living necessary for the child development". The third section of the same article indicates, "States Parties, in *accordance with national conditions and within their means*, shall take appropriate measures to assist the parents and others responsible for the child to implement this right and, *shall in case of need provide material assistance and support programs*, particularly with regard to *nutrition, clothing and housing*" (italics added).

We see how, in the first section, it is implicitly accepted that the children's standard of living corresponds to that of their parents, and that there are differences between children just like differences between adults. The second section, full of hedges, reduces the States space for intervention to "the necessary cases" and to resolving problems regarding the most essential questions, and addresses one of the characteristics of the residual and assistance model of welfare, in which benefits are not given directly to the children as individual persons, but to the family group as a whole.

This weakness in the State's role contrasts with the specific statements in the articles on compulsory education that follow. Article 28 of the Convention starts, "States Parties recognize the right of the child to education, and with a view to achieving this right progressively and on the basis of equal opportunity conditions, they *shall* specifically. . .".

This specifies the current agreement on children's social welfare: the State, acting as an interpreter and executor of social desirability, establishes and oversees the completion of the family's obligations, it substitutes them (exceptionally) and protects them (weakly), while simultaneously taking care of schooling, the elementary formation of the human capital.

Thus, the material welfare of children is linked to the economic potential of their families. Since the capacity to obtain an income is related, among other factors, with the life cycles of individuals, their value on the market and, in the case of family groups, the number of members capable of contributing with economic resources, the possibility for children to benefit from higher or lower family incomes will be in accordance to their parents' age, their parents' professional formation, how many people work at home and, likewise, the number of individuals with whom they have to share all possible income.

Because of the existence of all these inequalities both within homes and among individuals, the available income impacts on the possibilities of enjoying an adequate quality of life. At this point, it is best to agree that "the deep injustice in the distribution of wealth, a more limited labour market and one limited to precariousness and informality exert an impact mainly on that part of the population that has less resources" Scandizzo, (2001, p. 146, translated), with the inevitable result that a major part of the child population is located on the border of or below the levels that indicate poverty and social exclusion.

Besides all reasons due to the economic order, there are many other reasons from the social realm that shape and seal the deal between family and society for the minors' sustenance. The character of the relationship between parents and children involves a powerful element of cultural conservatism in which adult males are the main beneficiaries. The male person's authority prevails, and the subordination of the wife's and children's interests is deeply rooted in conservative tradition and supported from time to time by the waves of Puritanism or moralist thinking. The noninterventionist liberal vision tends to include the family in the area of the private sphere. This truly guarantees its liberty of reproduction and of the socialization of its offspring, but at the same time excludes and hinders the recognition of such a contribution to the material welfare of the community.

Currently, the family is gaining importance in the neoliberal model, assigning it a high degree of responsibility for the welfare of its members. As a result, it is becoming a key factor in the withdrawal of public policies and solutions for acquiring services in the market. On the opposite side (the universal welfare model), the different services and provisions have the goal of assuring the fulfilment of needs "from birth to death," guaranteeing at the same time the individuality and interdependence of the members of the family group (this is not an obstacle to children receiving services through their parents). Even though the different models have echoes in children's lives, it cannot be said that until now there has existed an approach that specifically considers the situation of the minors. Anyway, children's interest should be considered from here on. That fact should be supported both by justice reasons and for the welfare system sustainability.

To summarize, society receives new members who guarantee its future reproduction, but its contribution to cover their needs is scarce in terms of material and emotional well-being. The family orientation of the CRC is especially clear in those articles referring to provision rights, that is, rights that imply a budget. As a consequence of the implicit agreement between society, family and state, the children's situation depends on their parents' cultural and social position as well as on their capability to earn money in a segmented labour market. The more the parents are well positioned, the more children enjoy a *decent* standard of living. In contrast, the worse the situation of the parents, the worse is that of the children as well.

To modify this situation, the welfare state intervenes to distribute or redistribute social resources in order to reach a fair balance. The amount of resources involved is of major importance for children's well-being, as several studies and comparative research have shown (Bradshaw, 2007; Olk & Wintersberger, 2007; Wintersberger, 2006).

4 How Children Experience Their Well-Being

Decisions about children's well-being are broadly made in spaces that are usually closed to children. These are normally political decisions influenced by the interest of the majority of voters, be it on a national, regional or local level. As a consequence, we are speaking about a field of human activity in which children's rights have not been developed. As children's opinions do not count in this realm, social research seems to have no interest in exploring it. However, we can see a trend within the field of childhood studies to carry out research that coincides with the social spaces defined for children, such as the school, the kindergarten, the family or peer cultures.

In the study to be explained briefly below (Gaitán, 1999), we try to break with this tendency and approach the meaning of childhood for children themselves and see how they perceive themselves as children in a certain society along with their degree of satisfaction with their life and the arrangements provided for their own or others' well-being.

Twenty-two interviews were carried out with 10–14-year-old children living in the Madrid region. The topics of these children's discourses were classified into four categories:

1. The personal experience of being a child
2. Interpersonal relationships
3. Opinions about welfare state benefits
4. Specific difficulties in finding their own role and social space

Results showed that children are satisfied with their situation of being children and wish to stay/live in this society. Their main aspirations seem to be for more personal autonomy and better coverage of affective and material needs for every child. Regarding social policies, which are always a question of priorities, Spain seems to favour elderly and adult people, whereas children only receive benefits through their families. This disadvantage is breaking down with increasing education, and children are establishing their main exchanges with society through this. They understand education as a right, and are concerned about the quality of their studies along with the conditions and relations in the schools themselves.

Families seem to be effective in meeting children's needs, and even children belonging to the lower middle and lower classes with some economic difficulties expressed a high level of satisfaction with their family, and being able to share the good and bad things within it. Because they feel that the family provides means for

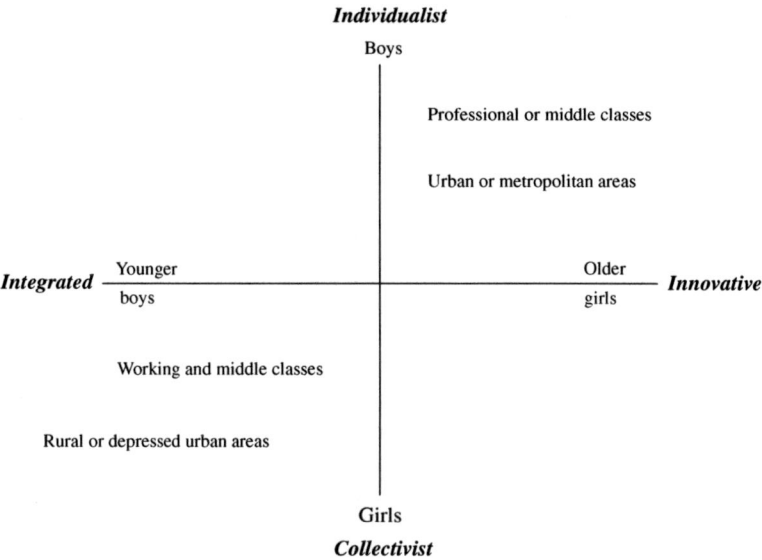

Fig. 1 Children's attitudes towards welfare benefits

them to be happy both in a material and/or affective sense, children are more linked to family affairs than to social aims.

With reference to the position that children adopt towards the external adult world, including the social welfare facilities, resources and protection provided by the state, four categories can be distinguished. These are represented by two axes in Fig. 1: vertical (from individual to collectivist position) and horizontal (from integrated to innovative).

Boys tend to be positioned in more individualistic and integrated areas, whereas girls seem to be located closer to innovation and collective affairs and problems. The integrated and collectivist positions are more common among children from the lower and middle classes or from rural and depressed environments. In contrast, individualistic and innovative attitudes are found among children from the professional or middle classes in urban and metropolitan areas.

A more recent international comparative study (UNICEF, 2007) confirms these interpretations to some extent. In terms of children's satisfaction with their lives, this study puts Spain in fifth place. That is not due to the level of material or educational satisfaction, but to *subjective well-being,* a concept that comprises satisfaction with their daily life in a warm family environment and with the family support they receive both in a material and emotional sense.

5 Conclusions

Briefly, it can be concluded that there is an implicit agreement conferring the main responsibility for the well-being of their children to parents. As a consequence, the welfare situation of children depends mainly on the cultural, social and economic position of their parents—with the implication that they will be as wealthy or as poor as their parents are.

In spite of the recognized *provision* rights for children, in general terms, states protect them weakly, or not as firmly as they should. The social images of children as dependents on their families sustain those kind of decisions or preferences that do not give priority to children.

A new contract providing priority to children is needed (Esping-Andersen, 2008). Such a contract should encompass the following aspects:

1. Social policies have to assure equal opportunities for all children.
2. The state has to guarantee a decent standard of living for them.
3. Society as a whole has to become responsible for children's well-being both in order to assert justice and as a necessity to ensure its own future survival.

References

Agathonos, H. (1993). Child protection within the convention on the rights of the child: A eulogy or a euphemism? In P. Heiliö, E. Lauronen, & M. Bardy (Eds.), *Politics of childhood and children at risk: Provision-protection-participation* (pp. 69–81). Vienna: European Centre for Social Welfare Policy and Research.

Bradshaw, J. (2007). Child benefit packages in 22 countries. In H. Wintersberger, L. Alanen, T. Olk, & J. Qvortrup (Eds.), *Childhood, generational order and the welfare state: Exploring children's social and economic welfare* (pp. 141–157). Odense: University Press of Southern Denmark.

Esping-Andersen, G. (2008), 'Childhood investments and skill formation,' *International Tax and Public Finance,* 15(1), 19–44

Gaitán, L. (1999). *El espacio social de la infancia. Los niños en el Estado del Bienestar.* Madrid: Comunidad de Madrid.

Gaitán, L. (2006). *Sociología de la infancia.* Madrid: Síntesis.

Heiliö, P., Lauronen, E., & Bardy, M. (1993). *Politics of childhood and children at risk. Provision-protection-participation.* Vienna: European Centre for Social Welfare Policy and Research.

Makrinioti, D. (1994). Conceptualization of childhood in a welfare state: A critical reappraisal. In J. Qvourtrup, M. Bardy, G. Sgritta, & H. Wintersberger (Eds.), *Childhood matters* (pp. 267–283). Aldershot: Avebury.

Marshall, T.H. 1950. Citizenship and Social Class and Other Essays. Cambridge: Cambridge University Press

Olk, T., & Wintersberger, H. (2007). Welfare state and generational order. In H. Wintersberger, L. Alanen, T. Olk, & J. Qvortrup (Eds.), *Childhood, generational order and the welfare state: Exploring children's social and economic welfare* (pp. 59–90). Odense: University Press of Southern Denmark.

Qvortrup, J. (1990). *Childhood as a social phenomenon: An introduction to a series of national reports* (Eurosocial Report 36). Vienna, Austria: European Centre for Social Welfare Policy and Research.

Recknagel, A. (2002). Déficits socio-culturales de la convención de los derechos del niño. *NATS, V*(9), 27–42.

Scandizzo, G. (2001). *Políticas públicas para la infancia. Una mirada desde los derechos.* Buenos Aires: Espacio Editorial.

UNICEF. (2007). *Child poverty in perspective: An overview of child well-being in rich countries* (Innocenti Report Card 7). Florence, Italy: UNICEF Innocenti Research Centre.

United Nations (1959). Declaration of the rights of the child. Geneva: The United Nations.

United Nations (1948). Universal Declaration of Human Rights. http://www.ohchr.org/EN/Issues/Pages/UDHRIndex.aspx

Wintersberger, H. (2006). Infancia y ciudadanía: el orden generacional del Estado de Bienestar. *Política y Sociedad, 43*(1), 81–103.

Children and Their Needs

Sabine Andresen and Stefanie Albus

1 Introduction

The discourse on the well-being of children reveals a variety of both implicit and explicit features that can be used as guidelines for judging whether children are doing well. In recent years, it has become increasingly popular to ask the children themselves about these features. As in happiness research with adults, the assumption is that every child, or every human being, is the one who knows best about her or his well-being, and which aspects of her or his life (family/social relations, material situation, possibilities of self-actualization, etc.) are relevant for her or him as an individual respondent in a specific situation (see Veenhoven, 2004, p. 20). However, even if studies now ascertain the general well-being of children by assessing subjective child satisfaction on the basis of categories specified by the researchers themselves and aggregate these to form indices (see Beisenherz, 2005, p. 165; Schneekloth & Leven, 2007, pp. 220–227), the background for choosing which are the relevant well-being factors still remains unclear, because of the lack of theoretical arguments in favour of selecting specific well-being dimensions.

During our search for suitable theoretical approaches to define and judge childhood well-being, we came across the need discourse. Until now, little attention has been paid to what an orientation towards the needs of children might contribute to research on their well-being. This represents the starting point for the present chapter in which we formulate relevant need theory approaches and plot their potential for a research that is oriented towards children, related to children and pays attention to their subjective abilities and their social framing conditions.

Defining human needs, their characteristics and the means to satisfy them has always been a challenging and demanding task for science, policy and practice. Formulating basic needs and perceiving and organizing paths and instruments for their satisfaction not only relate to fundamental ideas on human beings and what it is to be a human being but also involve the need to adopt a position with regard to the topic of justice and equality. Do we view children and adults predominantly as the

S. Andresen (✉)
Faculty of Educational Science, Bielefeld University, 33615 Bielefeld, Germany
e-mail: sabine.andresen@uni-bielefeld.de

S. Andresen et al. (eds.), *Children and the Good Life*, Children's Well-Being: Indicators and Research 4, DOI 10.1007/978-90-481-9219-9_5,
© Springer Science+Business Media B.V. 2010

human capital for a functioning work society? Or do we consider that the main task of society and politics is to focus on the well-being of each and every individual, because we recognize being human as an end in itself? Should all people be enabled to develop themselves personally and socially, or are support and promotion linked to specific conditions? Do we consider that the distribution of satisfiers should be regulated by the free market alone, or that it is essential for the state to engage in compensatory activities?

These are only a few of the relevant issues raised either explicitly or implicitly in the debate on needs. Further issues refer to the relation between the individuality and the universality of certain needs, and thereby also whether generation-specific differences need to be taken into account.

It seems meaningful to examine the needs of children separately, because a differentiation of life phases takes account of the current focus on relations between the generations. The formulation of children's needs reflects our view of childhood and the role assigned to children in our society. Analogue to the relation between our view of humanity and human needs, the decisive aspect when postulating children's needs is the paradigm of childhood on which studies are based. If children are conceived primarily as *adults-to-be*, other needs come to the fore than when childhood is conceived as an *independent life phase* in which children are assigned their own rights and recognized as possessing exclusive knowledge about what concerns them. Although it is meaningful to differentiate needs according to life phases, it is still important to grasp children's needs primarily as human needs. Children generally require other or additional means of satisfaction, and the status of individual needs may well shift with increasing age, but, nonetheless, the basic reference point is the human beingness of the child and, hence, the central hypothesis is that human needs serve as the starting point for children's needs.

The following section therefore starts by discussing approaches in need research that apply to all age groups. The third section addresses children's needs in order to clarify which specific demands they place on the family, the state and society. The final summary illustrates what the different need approaches have in common in order to provide a pragmatic basis for analysing the situation of children and adolescents in various contexts in light of need theory. In our opinion, such a broad-scale analysis of children's needs and their degree of satisfaction in different population groups offers the advantage of creating the preconditions for a fundamental reflection on childhood well-being and the further development of sociopolitical need-oriented measures from a perspective that transcends single disciplines and positions.

2 Theories of Human Needs

Both theoretical and empirical analyses of human needs can be found in a variety of disciplines, and this variety is reflected in the emphases taken by different approaches. The educational scientist Jutta Mägdefrau (2007) separates the approaches roughly by distinguishing between philosophical, political, sociological, psychological and educational lines of discussion in need research. Here, we can add need approaches that integrate a decisively practical concept in order to improve the living conditions of specific population groups or single individuals. These latter approaches have their roots in aid to developing countries or in critical social work. Although they refer in part to other (e.g. psychological) approaches, they do not fit completely into the above categories because of their pragmatic components. Therefore, we propose to distinguish them from the others by calling them sociopolitical need concepts.

In the following, we present the major psychological approaches and then refer to what we consider to be a useful sociological approach before finally discussing the Capabilities Approach formulated by Martha Nussbaum as an important theoretical framework for our work.

2.1 Psychological Need Concepts

Both the historical and the currently most dominant discussions in need research have their origins in psychology and specifically in motivation research (see Mägdefrau, 2007, p. 40). The drive underlying behaviour was the focus of various experiments in the newly developing science of psychology at the beginning of the twentieth century (see Hull, 1943; Woodworth, 1918). Several philosophical need theorists criticized these models of human behaviour for being mechanistic. This criticism cannot be rejected out of hand, because psychological need models are based particularly on cyclical concepts. With his dynamic and functional need concept, Kurt Lewin (1926) described this cycle as Tension—Satisfaction of need—Non-tension. The homeostatic model of need satisfaction can be viewed as a further development and differentiation of this tension cycle. In summary, the central motivation used to explain human behaviour here is the motivation to achieve balance.

Within both the psychological discourse and the interdisciplinary discussion, it has now become clear that this cyclical character is to be observed predominantly—if at all—only for vital needs such as hunger, thirst and sleep. For other groups of needs such as those for self-actualization, empirical research indicates more of a contrary dynamic (see Mägdefrau, 2007, p. 24). This makes it necessary to assume that experiencing self-actualization options or recognition by one's peers is unable to completely relieve the "tension state", because it is precisely the experience of self-actualization and recognition that supports the development of the need for these states of being. This is joined by the potential options of delaying the gratification of needs, suppressing tensions, or even sublimating or devaluing them (see Katz, 1933, p. 296). Nonetheless, the latter cannot overlook the fact that long-term frustration or nonsatisfaction can have far-reaching negative consequences such as deviant behaviour in children (see Katz, 1933). Both aspects point to the social components of need emphasized particularly by Henry Murray back in the 1930s. Katz (1933) had already labelled the mutability of needs, particularly the preferred means of satisfying them, with the terms "plasticity" and "periodicity", but Murray's analyses went further by considering the pressure that the environment exerts on the individual, "and indeed on the way in which needs are realized. This can occur in a manifest (alpha press) or a latent (beta press) way" (Mägdefrau, 2007, p. 41, translated).

The developmental aspect questions one prominent characteristic of needs: the universality of basic needs. The distinctions between need as a justified longing founded in human existence versus need as an arbitrary wanting (see Kamlah, 1972; Mallmann, 1980) seem to become blurred as soon as one considers their socialization. Against this background, one can fall back on the "basic needs approach" and the conceptual distinction between needs and means of realizing a need. This makes it possible to assume universal, anthropological needs that can claim to be valid across all cultures and individuals, while simultaneously taking account of the social nature of needs by pointing to the way the modes of need satisfaction are shaped by society. The reinterpretation of classical approaches against the background of this differentiation could be productive, and it defuses some of the elementary criticisms of the early psychological approaches of the twentieth century.

One of the first attempts in psychology to formulate a list of all relevant needs was performed by Murray, who finally compressed this into a list of over 20 needs (Murray, 1938). This included not only needs such as autonomy, play, recognition, care and eating, but also power and aggression. On closer inspection, two things stand out in Murray's list: *First*, it includes negative needs such as aggression, submission and rejection that are not to be found in other lists because of their predominantly humanistic view of society. *Second*, when so many terms are listed, we have to ask whether these are basic needs to be found in all cultures, or whether this list focuses specifically on the goals and socially moulded wishes that are recognized particularly in western societies.

This leads systematically to the question whether there is a hierarchy of needs, and bring us to the psychological need concept of Abraham Maslow. His pyramid of needs emphasizes their hierarchical aspect. Maslow assumed that there are needs that emerge only when basic needs have been met. The image of the pyramid visualizes the elitist background in Maslow's theory: "Higher" needs such as self-actualization are only attributed to people who possess the means to satisfy other "lower" needs. His classification of needs into deficiency and growth needs[1] took account of the criticism of a classical homoeostatic model and applied this productively (see Maslow, 1954). However, empirical studies have failed to support Maslow's hypotheses on a nested hierarchy of needs (see Wiswede, 1995). This leaves us with the relevant question of how far people in deficient conditions who are suffering from, for example, hunger, homelessness or violence feel the need for self-actualization if, for example, they have previously experienced its satisfaction at some time in their past.

---

[1] Maslow declared the deficiency needs to be physiological, safety, love, belongingness, respect (differentiated into self-respect and respect for others) and esteem. His growth needs, which he also called needs of being, included self-actualization that, nonetheless, cannot be satisfied completely (see the summary in Boeree, 2006).

Despite much criticism, Maslow's theory has influenced many of the need approaches in neighbouring disciplines. And although his hierarchy can be questioned both empirically and theoretically, his contribution has been to point so decisively to the significance of an existential basic provision of needs. Even in the current German discussion on the actualization of needs in children, it is appropriate not to lose sight of the satisfaction of their basic needs. At the present time, attention frequently focuses on the education aspect, and this is threatening to suppress discussion of the initial material situation within a child's family. The political discussions on school meals, the introduction of school benefits and the reintroduction of one-off grants for the children of those receiving state transfer funds represent positive counter-trends in this context that do not reduce the well-being of children to their institutional learning and care conditions.

Despite the indispensability of ensuring material and social basic needs through sociopolitical measures, it is necessary to avoid concentrating on the sufficient satisfaction of "deficiency" needs, because "growth" needs are also fundamental, as Maslow's critics have been able to show. As difficult as this may be due to limited resources, it is still necessary to ask how far the satisfaction of material, social and self-actualization needs can be promoted for all individuals.

Proceeding from an extended need perspective, another informative approach is that formulated by Edward Deci and Richard Ryan (2000). Their conceptual work focuses on three needs that are relevant for human well-being:

- Autonomy
- Competence
- Membership

They consider that none of these three needs can replace another; that is, all three have to be satisfied to promote mental health. Hence, they no longer consider physiological needs in their self-determination theory, because they view these as existential givens that have to be satisfied in order to ensure survival. Nonetheless, as a result, the modes of satisfying physiological needs and their potential influence on social and self-actualization needs remain in the darkness of non-scientific explanation—and clearly this can be viewed as a "blind spot" in this approach.

The main contribution of both psychologists is to emphasize that all action motives are no longer declared to be controlled by need per se or to be cognitive per se. Another major contribution from Deci and Ryan is that they not only extended the discourse on needs by differentiating between need-based action motivations and purely cognitive-based motivation, but also tempered the increasing dominance of cognitively oriented goal concepts in psychology during the final decades of the twentieth century by re-emphasising the importance of the need concept as well. Their need-based definition of psychological well-being makes it possible to analyse whether the action or the goal of the action serves to promote well-being by satisfying needs through the action, or whether the action goals are detached from need satisfaction.

Deci and Ryan not only assume the universal existence of needs in human beings but also stress the central role of social influences in the development of needs and their modes of satisfaction. The non-satisfaction of the three needs can have social consequences, because such need deprivation may express itself in illness and social disintegration (see Deci & Ryan, 2000).

2.2 Sociological Need Approaches

Alongside psychological approaches, a series of sociological concepts is also relevant for the present issue, not least because any discussion of the social dis-integration of persons also involves deficiencies in need satisfaction. An interesting approach here is the work of Karl-Otto Hondrich, who sees a conflictual two-sided relationship between needs and society that cannot be resolved. While Hondrich assumes that needs are conveyed by society, he rejects the idea that all persons nec-essarily adapt themselves optimally to the possibilities of need satisfaction their society allows them. This means that the individual is always in a potentially conflictual relationship with social authorities (see Hondrich, 1973). For exam-ple, surveys on satisfaction have shown that dissatisfaction with the opportunities allowed does not always show a linear relationship to the degree of need satisfac-tion, but that the outlook for future improvement impacts decisively on whether or not one is satisfied with one's current need situation (see Mägdefrau, 2007, p. 39).

The phenomenon of adaptation or of adaptive preferences is frequently addressed in the need discussion (see Kahn, 1972; Nussbaum, 2000; Sen, 1985). In both need research and policy making, this leads to the question regarding which predictive power surveys on satisfaction possess, and which influence these should have on policy making. Indeed, if one takes the critical finding seriously that the feeling of satisfaction is extremely susceptible to bias and manipulation, and that satisfaction can also be viewed as an expression of resignation and pessimism about the future, then promoting people's satisfaction would seem to be a questionable goal for policy measures. If the intention is to actually improve the need situation, it would seem advisable to take an (additional) orientation towards objective indicators (such as the actual availability of certain means to satisfaction) when evaluating the success of social policies.

Regarding this problem of adaptation, the Finnish sociologist Erik Allardt has also delivered useful proposals for a systematic analysis of life conditions from the need perspective. Allardt calls "Having," "Loving" and "Being" the three central categories of needs. Without their satisfaction, human beings cannot survive or avoid suffering, cannot enter into relationships with other human beings and cannot avoid alienation (see Allardt, 1993, pp. 89–93). Allardt's criticism of traditional research on welfare in the social sciences is that central aspects of human well-being, and thereby also satisfaction of needs, are examined uniquely and one-sidedly in terms of mean scores. As useful as such data are, they tell us little about whether (and, if so, how many) people can even begin to satisfy the above-mentioned needs. Referring to Johann Galtung, Allardt therefore proposes defining a threshold value to provide

Table 1 Different indicators for research on living conditions

	Objective indicators	Subjective indicators
Having (Material and impersonal needs)	1. Objective measures of the level of living and environmental conditions	4. Subjective feelings of dissatisfaction/satisfaction with living conditions
Loving (Social needs)	2. Objective measures of relationships with other people	5. Unhappiness/happiness— subjective feelings about social relations
Being (Needs for personal growth)	3. Objective measures of people's relation to (a) society (b) nature	6. Subjective feelings of alienation/personal growth

Source: Allardt (1993, p. 93)

a minimum score for the need satisfaction of every single individual in a specific society (see Allardt, 1993; Galtung, 1975).

Allardt overcomes the problem of subjectivity and objectivity by proposing that one should not only use objective indicators but also survey subjective appraisals and feelings. An overview of these indicators is given in Table 1.

2.3 Needs from the Perspective of the Capabilities Approach

Deciding on a minimum threshold for need satisfaction also requires a definition of the "good life". Therefore, this is the point at which we wish to discuss the social-philosophical approach of Martha Nussbaum and her interest in true human needs. Martha Nussbaum has summarized the central features of being human on the basis of Aristotelian premises and integrated them into the following list that she calls the "Capabilities Approach" (Albus, Andresen, Fegter, & Richter, 2009):

1. *Life*: Being able to live to the end of a human life of normal length
2. *Bodily health*: Being able to have good health, particularly in terms of adequate nourishment, shelter, reproductive health and mobility
3. *Bodily integrity*: Being able to avoid unnecessary pain and experience joy; to move freely from place to place; to have one's bodily boundaries treated as sovereign
4. *Senses, imagination, and thought*: Being able to use one's senses to imagine, think and reason
5. *Emotions*: Being able to have attachments to things and people, to love, to grieve, to experience longing and gratitude
6. *Practical reason*: Being able to form a conception of the good and engage in critical reflection about planning one's life

7. *Affiliation*: Being able to live with and towards others; to enter various forms of familial and social relationships *and* having the social bases of self-respect
8. *Other species*: Being able to live with concern for and in relation to animals, plants and the world of nature
9. *Play*: Being able to laugh, to play and to enjoy recreational activities
10. *Control over one's environment*: Being able to live one's own life and not somebody else's; participation, rights and being able to hold property in terms of real opportunity (Nussbaum, 2000)

Whether all these aspects of human lifestyle are perceived as needs by all individuals in an identical way is of only secondary importance according to the Capabilities perspective. Every individual has to decide which abilities actually are realized; that is, nobody is compelled to realize these human actualization potentials. What is far more important is the provision of the real freedoms to shape one's life according to one's own conception of the good (see Sen, 2001). Real freedoms in this context are more than just the distribution of resources and less than the need satisfaction that actually occurs: They are the possibilities that the individual could realize through the available structural resources, individual abilities and social rights—should he or she wish to (see Otto & Ziegler, 2006).[2]

The focus on real freedoms represents one central point in which the "Capabilities Approach" differs from the "Basic Needs Approach" (see Alkire, 2002; Sen, 1984). The Basic Needs Approach is particularly prominent in aid to developing countries. Despite its successes in empirically mapping conflicts over limited means of satisfying needs (see Mägdefrau, 2007, p. 69), this approach has been criticized particularly for its practical consequence of potentially reproducing inequality. For example, back in 1980, Galtung already pointed out that due to the focus on the potential damage of non-satisfaction and the possibilities of distinguishing between means of satisfaction, aid to the disadvantaged tends to concentrate on satisfying material needs, because the damage caused by their non-satisfaction is more apparent than that due to the non-satisfaction of immaterial needs. Hence, to help as efficiently as possible, a hierarchy of means of satisfaction is generated in which the means of satisfaction assigned to the disadvantaged are

---

[2] To give a simple example, the opportunity to be suitably nourished is given when enough food is available that an individual can also tolerate and is capable of eating—a steak would probably not meet this criterion for a person with no teeth. Therefore, in this case, the provision of a real freedom to nourish oneself appropriately would involve not only the availability of food but also appropriate dental care and the provision of false teeth. It also has to be considered whether the consumption of the available food violates cultural norms or values—it may be decisive here whether the piece of meat is beef, pork or lamb. When related to the lifeworld of children in Germany, the philosophy of the Capabilities Approach has to be examined in terms of extracurricular provisions in sports clubs and the like. However, the mere implementation of services does not suffice. Any examination of the actual possibilities that single children have to take advantage of these provisions has to take account of their mobility, their other obligations, whether their parents can pay club fees and so forth. However, at the end of the day, whether children actually do take up an offer by a club is less decisive. In light of their right to self-determination and participation, this is a decision that they must be left to make by themselves.

allocated by the satisfiers preferred by the elite (see, for a critical account, Galtung, 1980). In a similar way, the scientific search for a necessary minimum standard is considered to be at risk of exhausting its practical efforts in attaining this standard, but not in going beyond this. In view of such limitations, the utility of the Basic Needs Approach outside developmental aid in poor countries is questionable (see Sen, 1984).

A further criticism is that the approach focuses too strongly on the means of satisfaction and thereby ignores the individual possibilities of using these goods for one's own purposes (see Sen, 1984). Nonetheless, Alkire (2002, p. 168) has pointed out that this criticism is also shared by supporters of the Basic Needs Approach, making it necessary to assume that this limitation is not necessarily due to the approach itself but due to its pragmatic application in the practice of developmental aid.

3 Focusing Research on the Needs of Children

Recent years have also seen an increased integration of the clients into the need discourse and need definitions, and this has extended to research on children's needs as well. Asking children about their needs and their possibilities of satisfying them is a challenging undertaking (see Ben-Arieh, 2005). However, it can be viewed as empirical social research's contribution to complying with the children's right to participation. Which needs are relevant for a good childhood from the perspective of children? Interestingly, the needs they express do not differ spectacularly from the classifications of needs worked out from the scientific, from the adult perspective. This reveals that childhood studies are well advised not to assume any principal alienation between children and adults. Analyses of the results of a survey of 11,000 British 14- to 16-year-olds produced the following factors for a good childhood (see Children's Society, 2006):

- Qualitatively valuable relationships (love, care and respect)
  - Family
  - Friends
  - Community
- Freedoms and limits
  - Leisure time and recreation
  - Local environment
- Learning/Education
  - Attitudes
- Security
  - Money
- Health

Interesting findings can also be found in a study by Biggeri, Libanora, Mariani, and Menchini (2006) who surveyed 105 children and adolescents aged 11–17 years during a conference on child labour. The majority of these under-age respondents came from developing and threshold countries and possessed personal experience of child labour. When asked which possibilities of self-actualization they considered to be existentially important for children and adolescents in general, the majority reported the following factors:

- Love and care
- Physical integrity and security
- Education
- Leisure time and relaxation
- For adolescents: Participation

Fattore, Mason and Watson's (2007) study on the conceptions of well-being from the children's perspective also performed an explorative survey of the wishes and needs of children and adolescents. Responses from 126 children and adolescents aged 8–15 years revealed the following emphases:

- Autonomy and agency
- Protection and security
- Development of an identity (recognition, optimism, self-esteem)
- Material resources
- Environment and accommodation (space, living environment/leisure-time options)
- Activity and productivity

In contrast to this, the two physicians T. Berry Brazelton and Stanley I. Greenspan have assembled a systematic synopsis of the special needs of children from their professional perspective[3] and looked for ways in which, and to which extent, these needs can best be satisfied (see Brazelton & Greenspan, 2008). Based on their clinical and scientific experience as either a paediatrician or a child psychiatrist and with reference to several relevant studies, they found that the predominant needs of children are for,

- Consistent loving relationships
- Physical integrity, security and regulation
- Experiences tailored to individual differences
- Experiences appropriate to their level of development
- Limits and structures

---

[3] In German-speaking countries, the educational scientist Annegret Werner (2006) has also compiled a list of purely child-specific needs. Her list covers the need for subsistence, social attachment and bonds, and growth. The selection is based on developmental psychology and has taken its place within the debate on child protection (in the handbook *Kindeswohlgefährdung nach §1666 BGB und Allgemeiner Sozialer Dienst* [ASD]).

- Stable supportive communities and cultural continuity
- Safeguarding the future

They view the satisfaction of these needs as a task for society as a whole and as an absolute necessity. Looking at the United States, Brazelton and Greenspan diagnose less understanding on how to support families efficiently than other cultures despite its wealth, and a great risk that children will have to pay a terrible price for this later in the form of drug addiction, antisocial behaviour and violence (Brazelton & Greenspan, 2008, p. 10). Despite the obvious differences in the two welfare systems, there is a clear need for critical reflection on whether the major fields of conflict addressed by Brazelton and Greenspan are also to be found in Germany and other European countries. Aspects such as the continuously growing demands on both parents to be highly successful caregivers as well as highly productive in working life, and the frequently inadequate private and public possibilities of support are everyday topics in, for example, German discussions in politics, science and society.

Brazelton and Greenspan do not just explain to parents how they can ensure and promote the well-being of their children. They also formulate recommendations regarding the quality of publicly organized childcare. This relates satisfying the needs of children explicitly to the organizational measures of childcare. Ranging from the ratio of children to caregivers to the reimbursement of these caregivers and their training, Brazelton and Greenspan clarify how these factors impact on the consistency and quality of the relation between child and caregiver.

Consistent loving relationships play a central role in Brazelton and Greenspan's need concept. They form the starting point for the feeling of security, the ability to learn self-regulation and the further emotional and cognitive development of the child. This finding is also revealed in an explorative study on child poverty in Germany, although a further aspect also proves to be relatively important here: avoiding shame and shaming (Andresen & Fegter, 2009). One feature of relationships that promotes development and security is, in general, "reciprocal interactions" that require both continuity and sensitivity from the adult caregiver while taking care to avoid shaming children and their families—particularly when they are living in socially precarious conditions.

With regard to the general discussion on need theory, it should be recalled once more that the so-called needs for growth and self-actualization are linked inseparably to the need for social belongingness. Without a consistent, attentive and empathic reference person, according to Brazelton and Greenspan (2008, pp. 39–40), children have no chance to control their feelings and perceive themselves as part of the social fabric.

In view of these major demands on those caring for babies and infants, we have to ask who is in any way qualified for this task. Here, Brazelton and Greenspan predominantly talk about parents (paying particular attention to mothers[4]), but

---

[4] At this point, it becomes clear that the two authors' recommendations are based on a limited critical and reflective attitude towards their own cultural background and the hegemonic strivings of the

because they also admit that specific reasons prevent round-the-clock care by parents, they include further caregivers in their recommendations. The two authors take a closer look at the framing conditions in day nurseries and toddler groups. Based on their own observations and the contemporary state of research, they conclude that this form of care is not organized optimally in the United States, and is therefore of questionable effectiveness. During the further course of child development, the preconditions for individual, developmentally appropriate educational experiences are also of major importance. Brazelton and Greenspan call for teaching in schools to take the individuality of children into account, and they criticize the pressure to succeed imposed on children. In addition, they recommend smaller learning groups or classes containing 12–15 students (see Brazelton & Greenspan, 2008, pp. 189–190), assuming that the current class size of 25–30 children systematically impedes individual interaction between teachers and their students. School stress and continuous mental overload frequently lead children to become disturbed and diagnosed as being in need of treatment by teachers, parents, physicians and so forth. Brazelton and Greenspan (2008, p. 21) point out that there is an observable trend to treat children with drugs that will enable them to handle demands again as quickly as possible.

An alternative approach to that sketched above is to look at what needs to be satisfied from the perspective of children's rights. With their three emphases on rights to protection; to care; and to culture, information and participation, the United Nations Convention on the Rights of the Child reflects the need debate presented above.

The UNICEF Committee for monitoring implementation of and compliance with children's rights has also specified the following principles of the Convention on the Rights of the Child as being relevant for monitoring children's living conditions and their legal statutes:

- *The principle of non-discrimination (Article 2 of the Convention on the Rights of the Child).*
  This specifies that statistics on a national or similar level do not possess sufficient predictive power: indicators must reflect the degree of compliance with the rights of specific population groups—particularly those of the most disadvantaged in order to evaluate these and dismantle inequalities.
- The *principle of the best interests of the child (Article 3).*
  In all cases, the choice of indicators should reflect the perspective of the Convention on the Rights of the Child that grants priority to the child's best

---

(male) educated middle class. The emphatic recommendation for or against specific means of satisfaction (e.g. mothers or parents as preferred reference persons, the implicit criticism of technology at certain points, etc.)—which promise behavioural certainty and initially present themselves as a welcome starting point for political and practical reforms—conceal the fact that preferences for specific means of satisfaction vary both historically and culturally. Likewise, the authors contradict their own beliefs—that the needs of every child differ individually—by formulating generalized but very concrete recommendations.

interests. This principle is also useful for testing how far budgeting gives priority to children and their rights.

- *The principle of respect for the views of children and their right of participation (Articles 12–15)*
  This principle defines children not as passive receivers but as agents to be included actively in decisions that impact on their lives.
- *The principle of the child's right to life and development (Article 6)*
  This principle covers the entire range of the child's rights to develop her or his full potential, starting with the satisfaction of the needs in regard to health, nutrition and education in order to promote personal and social development. The well-being of children is not only the responsibility of the family and the state but just as much the responsibility of the complete society of nations (UNICEF, 1998, p. 7).

The list of principles clarifies how close relations can be between scientific need concepts, national negotiation products and sociopolitical measures.

4 Need Theories and the Well-Being of Children: Provisional Conclusion

Our analysis of the different scientific approaches to need reveals several universal aspects that need to be taken into account when discussing children's (and all people's) needs:

- *Needs are supraindividual.*
  They are more than just individual wishes. Most of the approaches presented assume that needs are universal. And even approaches that are critical of universalism generally assume a justified desire that is reconcilable with socially acceptable patterns of legitimisation or with culturally anchored images of humanity.
- *Needs are normative constructs.*
  Needs are not abstract, but express themselves in a concrete and individually perceivable state of tension. Whether the reason for this state is called a need (and not a wish etc.) depends on the observer's view of humanity and her or his conception of what a person or child needs to be a person or child.
- *Needs, or more precisely the paths to their satisfaction, are shaped by conditions in society.*
  On the one hand, socially mediated preferences form in the selection of means of need satisfaction. On the other hand, individuals depend on other persons to satisfy their needs. The central question in this context can be formulated as follows: How far do the structures in society lead to different or similar strategies of need satisfaction, and how far do the structures in society allow individuals to satisfy their own needs?

- *Needs, or more precisely the possibilities of their satisfaction, may differ individually.*

  Differences in the possibilities of satisfying needs are based on the physical and mental possibilities and limitations of individuals as well as on their position in society and their integration within social communities. The interdependence of these different factors also explains the need for a comprehensive analytical approach to fighting need deprivation.
- *Needs, or more precisely the way in which they are satisfied, vary across the life course.*

  In the different stages of development (infancy, childhood, adolescence, ... old age), human beings vary in how far they depend on external help to satisfy their needs. In addition, the recognition of needs relates to the socially constructed and legitimised concept of the specific life phase.

Despite these characteristics, central need categories can be singled out on the basis of the need concepts presented above, and these need to be taken into account in the discussion on the well-being of children in the sense of striving towards an adequate satisfaction of their needs (see Fig. 1).

Any appropriate empirical assessment of these central categories must consider not only objective indicators such as the presence of material resources, available relationships and education programmes but also the subjective attitudes of children and adolescents towards their life circumstances.

Moreover, when it comes to the state of need, it is essential to perform analyses that are sensitive to inequality in order not only to recognize socioeconomic or class-specific preferences but also, and above all, to make absolute-need poverty visible and thereby accessible to intervention.

In the fight against precarious need states, we should never forget that disadvantaged children and adolescents also have a right to participation, and that their integration into decision-making processes may well represent a first step towards satisfying their need for recognition and self-determination.

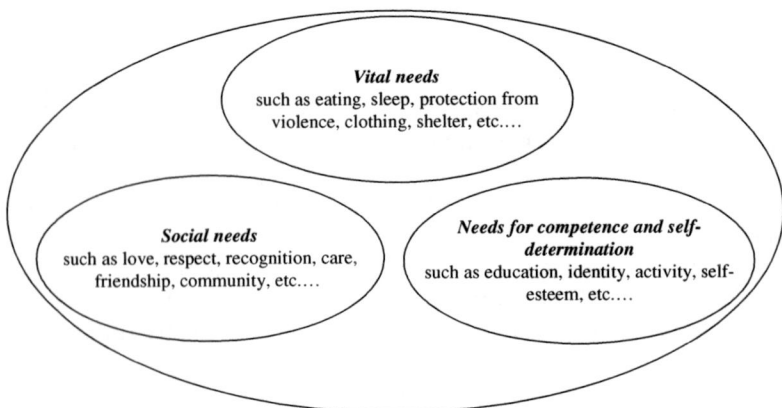

Fig. 1 Major categories in the need discourse

References

Albus, S., Andresen, S., Fegter, S., & Richter, M. (2009). Wohlergehen und das „gute Leben" in der Perspektive von Kindern. Das Potenzial das Capability Approach für die Kindheitsforschung. *Zeitschrift für Soziologie der Erziehung und Sozialisation, 29*(4), 346–358.

Alkire, S. (2002). *Valuing freedoms: Sen's capability approach and poverty reduction.* New York: Oxford University Press.

Allardt, E. (1993). Having, loving, being: An alternative to the Swedish model of welfare research. In M. C. Nussbaum & A. K. Sen (Eds.), *The quality of life* (pp. 88–94). Oxford: Clarendon.

Andresen, S., & Fegter, S. (2009). *Spielräume sozial benachteiligter Kinder. Bepanthen Kinderarmutsstudie. Eine ethnographische Studie zu Kinderarmut in Hamburg und Berlin.* Preliminary final report. Bielefeld University, Germany.

Beisenherz, G. (2005). Wie wohl fühlst du dich? Kindliche Persönlichkeit und Umwelt als Quelle von Wohlbefinden und Unwohlsein bei Grundschulkindern. In C. Alt (Ed.), *Kinderleben – Aufwachsen zwischen Familie, Freunden und Institutionen. Band 1: Aufwachsen in Familien* (pp. 157–186). Wiesbaden: VS-Verlag.

Ben-Arieh, A. (2005). Where are the children? Children's role in measuring and monitoring their well-being. *Social Indicators Research, 74*(3), 573–596.

Biggeri, M., Libanora, R., Mariani, S., & Menchini, L. (2006). Children conceptualizing their capabilities: Results of a survey conducted during the first children's world congress on child labour. *Journal of Human Development, 7*(1), 59–83.

Boeree, C. G. (2006). *Persönlichkeitstheorien: Abraham Maslow* (D. Wiesner Trans.). http://www.social-psychology.de/do/PT_maslow.pdf. Accessed March 10, 2009.

Brazelton, T. B., & Greenspan, S. I. (2008). *Die sieben Grundbedürfnisse von Kindern. Was jedes Kind braucht, um gesund aufzuwachsen, gut zu lernen und glücklich zu sein.* Beltz, Weinheim, Germany.

Children's Society. (2006). *Good childhood? A question for our times.* A National Inquiry. Summary of Launch Report. http://www.childrenssociety.org.uk/resources/documents/good%20childhood/Good_Childhood_Inquiry_launch_report_5830_full.pdf. Accessed March 10, 2009.

Deci, E. L., & Ryan, R. M. (2000). The "what" and "why" of goal pursuits: Human needs and the self-determination of behavior. *Psychological Inquiry, 11*(4), 27–268.

Fattore, T., Mason, J., & Watson, E. (2007). Children's conceptualisation(s) of their well-being. *Social Indicators Research, 80*(1), 5–29.

Galtung, J. (1975). Measuring world development I. *Alternatives, 1,* 131–158.

Galtung, J. (1980). The basic needs approach. In K. Lederer (Ed.), *Human needs: A contribution to the current debate* (pp. 55–125). Cambridge, MA: Oelgeschlager, Gunn & Hain.

Hondrich, K.-O. (1973). Bedürfnisorientierung und soziale Konflikte – zur theoretischen Begründung eines Forschungsprogramms. *Zeitschrift für Soziologie, 2*(3), 263–281.

Hull, C. L. (1943). *Principles of behavior: An introduction to behavior theory.* New York: Appleton-Century-Crofts.

Kahn, R. L. (1972). The meaning of work: Interpretation and proposals for measurement. In A. Campbell & P. E. Converse (Eds.), *The human meaning of social change* (pp. 159–204). New York: Russel Sage.

Kamlah, W. (1972). *Philosophische Anthropologie. Sprachkritische Grundlegung und Ethik.* Mannheim: Bibliographisches Institut.

Katz, D. (1933). Zur Grundlegung einer Bedürfnispsychologie. *Zeitschrift für Psychologie, 129,* 292–304.

Lewin, K. (1926). *Vorsatz, Wille und Bedürfnis.* Berlin: Springer.

Mägdefrau, J. (2007). *Bedürfnisse und Pädagogik. Eine Untersuchung an Hauptschulen.* Bad Heilbrunn: Julius Klinkhardt.

Mallmann, C. A. (1980). Society, needs, and rights: A systematic approach. In K. Lederer (Ed.), *Human needs: A contribution to the current debate* (pp. 227–232). Cambridge, MA: Oelgeschlager, Gunn & Hain.

Maslow, A. H. (1954). *Motivation and personality*. New York: Harper.

Murray, H. (1938). *Explorations in personality*. New York: Oxford University Press.

Nussbaum, M. C. (2000). *Woman and human development*. Cambridge, UK: Cambridge University Press.

Otto, H.-U., & Ziegler, H. (2006). Capabilities and education. *Social Work & Society, 4*(2), 269–287. http://www.socwork.net/2006/2/articles/ottoziegler/ottoziegler.pdf. Accessed December 03, 2008.

Schneekloth, U., & Leven, I. (2007). Wünsche, Ängste und erste politische Interessen. In World Vision Deutschland e.V. (Ed.), *Kinder in Deutschland 2007. 1. World Vision Kinderstudie* (pp. 201–225). Frankfurt a. M.: Fischer.

Sen, A. K. (1984). *Resources, values and development*. Oxford: Basil Blackwell.

Sen, A. K. (1985). *Commodities and capabilities*. Amsterdam: North Holland.

Sen, A. K. (2001). *Development as freedom*. New York: Oxford University Press.

UNICEF. (1998). *Indicators for global monitoring of child rights*. Summary report and background papers of the International meeting February 9–12 in Geneva, Switzerland. UNICEF, New York. http://kmsodd.wfp.org/managerdoc/paystheme/Regional%20Bureau%20OMD/Programme%20Support%20Unit/Nutrition/UNICEF%20INDICATORS%201999.pdf Accessed February 05, 2009.

Veenhoven, R. (2004). *Subjective measures of well-being*. (Discussion Paper No. 2004/07). Helsinki, Finland: UNU-WIDER. http://www.wider.unu.edu/publications/working-papers/discussion-papers/2004/en_GB/dp2004-007/. Accessed January 15, 2008.

Werner, A. (2006). Was brauchen Kinder, um sich altersgemäß zu entwickeln. In H. Kindler, S. Lillig, H. Blüml, T. Meysen, & A. Werner (Eds.), *Handbuch Kindeswohlgefährdung nach § 1666 und Allgemeiner Sozialer Dienst (ASD)* (pp. 131–134). Munich: Verlag Deutsches Jugendinstitut. http://db.dji.de/asd/F013_Werner_lv.pdf. Accessed March 10, 2009.

Wiswede, G. (1995). *Einführung in die Wirtschaftspsychologie* (2nd ed.). Munich: E. Reinhardt.

Woodworth, R. S. (1918). *Dynamic psychology*. New York: Columbia University Press.

Part II
The Capability Approach and Research on Children

Zoé Clark and Franziska Eisenhuth

1 Introduction

Within this introduction, we shall briefly relate some ideas from New Social Childhood Studies (NSCS)—as one currently dominant way of thinking within childhood studies—to the analytical focus suggested by the Capabilities Approach (CA) and, in particular, Martha Nussbaum.

At least two lines of argument within NSCS can be addressed from a capabilities perspective. We start by outlining a general theoretical problem that accompanies a specific concept of the child favoured within NSCS, and then describe how this theoretical problem implies methodological problems, particularly within action research. Currently this research approach is often combined with the CA in research projects on children. After examining these problems, we shall outline the conditions under which NSCS and the CA can be brought together productively.

2 The Concept of the Child Within NSCS: Problems from a Capabilities Perspective

In the field of childhood studies, we are referring to New Social Childhood Studies (NSCS). NSCS represents a paradigm that is acquiring a growing influence within childhood studies. The term covers various, mainly sociological fields of research, in which the common factor is their claim to develop a new, social constructivist perspective on childhood.

One main suggestion of the NSCS is to focus on children's current life situations instead of deeming a child as "on her/his way to humanness" and "in a state of becoming" (Qvortrup, 2005, p. 3)—a criticism directed towards the conventional

Z. Clark (✉)
Research School Education and Capabilities, Bielefeld University, 33615 Bielefeld, Germany
e-mail: zoe.clark@uni-bielefeld.de

child sciences of developmental psychology and socialisation theory. It is especially one track within NSCS, focusing on childhood as a part of social structure, that links this claim to concentrate on children's well-being instead of on their well-becoming with a specific concept of children as competent agents. Children are taken as 'full members of society' (ibid.) who contribute to its reproduction and should therefore be granted equal rights with adults.

This is a rather clear way of positioning oneself in the conceptual debate on how autonomous children are versus how dependent they are. Taking a position within this debate implies an answer to the question whether that which a child expresses as his or her desires is tantamount to the best interest of the child. On the basis of an analytical distinction between subjective preferences and an 'objectively' defined well-being of the child, it can be said that NSCS risk overemphasising children's perspectives and romanticising the agency of children. Reducing justice for young people to subjective well-being assumes that they are fully able to ascertain how their own life situation is embedded into the social structure (Gallacher & Gallagher, 2008). This assumption ignores the fact that people adapt their preferences and (future) aspirations to their current life situation. Nussbaum (2007, p. 73) argues that focusing on subjective well-being runs the risk of perpetuating social inequality. Also, individuals in deprived life situations tend to adapt their preferences to their limited possibilities to live a valuable life. A position that welcomes children's desires and aspirations affirmatively as an isolated metric for justice faces a risk of becoming cynical.

3 Action Research with Children: Problems from a Capabilities Perspective

This risk of romanticising children's agency is, from our point of view, reflected in methodological problems within NSCS. The methodological rediscovery of action research is closely related to the paradigmatic shift accompanying the NSCS.

Within NSCS and participatory action research on children, the dominant notion of the child as a research subject is criticised in two ways:

1. On the one hand, the NSCS paradigm implies an intrinsic ethical argument for the redistribution of intergenerational power relationships and a democratisation of the research process. Adult research on children is criticised as a non-democratic way of producing knowledge. Accordingly, it is concluded that young people should, instead, be empowered as participants within the whole process of research, and hence be recognised as competent and autonomous agents.
2. On the other hand, there is an instrumental technical argument related to the quality of the data. Beyond the ethical issues, it is assumed within the paradigm of action research that the only ones who can produce authentic knowledge about

children are the children themselves. In other words, research should 'use' the knowledge of children in order to produce 'good', that is, 'authentic' data.[1]

Central questions that should be addressed in order to gain a 'complete picture of human beings in their present life … that values them as legitimate members of their community and society' are, for example, the following '(1) What are children doing? (2) What do children need? (3) What do children have? (4) What do children think and feel? (5) To whom or what are children connected and related? And (6) What do children contribute?' (Ben-Arieh, 2005, p. 577).

4 A Productive Combination of Childhood Research and a Capabilities Perspective

From the perspective of the Capabilities Approach (CA), there are certain restraints on merely doing research on how people assess their own situation, what they do and what their contributions are. People's life situations, aspirations and values are not only an outcome of—and thus within the responsibility of—individual preferences and abilities. It is not enough to ask people what they need in order to give them a democratic voice. What they utter as needs should always be analysed as being embedded in social structures.

The general yardstick for just conditions within the CA is formulated as the ethical equality of each and every human, independent of their abilities and of the question whether they contribute anything or not (see Nussbaum, 2007, p. 66 ff.). Therefore, the CA draws an important distinction between functionings and capabilities. While functionings are the current doings and beings of persons, capabilities mean the real freedom of people to realise the life they have reason to value. Based on this fundamental distinction, research within the context of the CA should focus on what the individual capability set looks like, including both obstacles and opportunities. Accordingly, research on children would not address current doings and beings of the young people as subjects of research, but focus on their capabilities to lead a full human life that allows them to develop their full human potential, without any need to assess their contribution in order to legitimise their full membership.

Beyond this general perspective on personhood, the CA does not yet have much to offer with regard to a concept of childhood and justice in the context of growing up. The currently dominant perception of the CA results in a quite contrary positioning of the concept of the child between the poles of autonomy and dependency compared to that of NSCS. It is striking that whereas a capability perspective in

---

[1] Why children are treated as a population of their own with age-specific interests and how to deal with other lines of difference like class, gender or 'race', in order to generate so-called authentic data remain largely unquestioned.

general argues for a latitude of individual choices (which is implied in the notion of capabilities), it seems to be largely commonsense that a child's freedom of choice has to be restricted in favour of developing future capabilities. Here, the CA tends to overemphasise the best interests of the child, understood as objectively determinable well-being independent of subjective well-being.

But even if Nussbaum and Sen widely exclude children and tend to apply a functionings rather than a capabilities approach when talking about them, we still argue that the CA can be applied to childhood studies in a very productive way. We claim that the same metric of human dignity applied to adults should also be addressed to children, even though it might need to be specified in a certain age-dependent way.[2]

Taking its ethically individualistic perspective seriously, the CA offers what the NSCS demands, that is, an opportunity to recognise the well-being and the life standard of children as individual persons. Hence, children are not simply one part of a family, but deemed own entities of well-being and dignity. Such an understanding of the CA answers the demands expressed by the NSCS that childhood should not be sacrificed to later stages of adulthood, should not be reduced to a stage of transition and incompleteness.

Still, it has to be said that while the notion of well-becoming for young people is sharply criticised and rejected within the NSCS as being future-oriented, one main project within the CA is to define human development or human flourishing and hence becoming 'truly human'. But this notion of development is not to be misunderstood as a psychological term for forming an identity at an early age. The notion of human development within the CA is initially neither age-specific nor related to the development of a predefined good identity, but refers to the freedom of each and every person to develop the doings and beings he or she has reason to value in order to form a good life. Therefore, this terminology of development does not necessarily reduce and sacrifice childhood to later stages of adulthood, even though it always at least implies a future-oriented aspect.

From our point of view, it would be wise to use the Capabilities Approach as a frame for a theory of justice for young people that includes the current well-being of children in order to not sacrifice this stage of life to later adulthood, without ignoring the instrumental role childhood plays in the context of the intergenerational reproduction of social inequality. On the one hand, current capabilities should play a role for children, without denying their competencies to make choices; but, on the other hand, the unequal distribution of functionings related to future freedoms should not be forgotten either. In this understanding, a capabilities perspective can contribute to theoretical reflections on childhood, and, in turn, certain assumptions within New Social Childhood Studies can provide a fruitful reflection on the concept of the child within the Capabilities Approach.

---

[2]In order to outline such specifications, it appears to be very reasonable to include young people as sources of information, as Ben-Arieh, amongst others, has suggested.

References

Ben-Arieh, A. (2005). Where are the children? Children's role in measuring and monitoring their well-being. *Social Indicators Research, 74*, 573–596.

Gallacher, L.-A., & Gallagher, M. (2008). Methodological immaturity in childhood research? Thinking through 'participatory methods'. *Childhood, 15*, 499–516.

Nussbaum, M. (2007). *Frontiers of justice: Disability, nationality, species membership.* Cambridge, MA: Harvard University Press.

Qvortrup, J. (2005). Varieties of childhood. In J. Qvortrup (Ed.), *Studies in modern childhood: Society, agency, culture* (pp. 1–20). New York: Palgrave Macmillan.

The Capability Approach and Research on Children: Capability Approach and Children's Issues

Mario Biggeri, Jérôme Ballet, and Flavio Comim

1 Capability Approach and Children: A Review of Empirical Analyses

Although the Capability Approach and human development research is often concerned with the deprivation of children's capabilities and functionings, few studies have examined children's capabilities.[1] However, in this new field of research, there is already a small number of recent empirical studies that are worth mentioning. In this section, we review all the papers and field researches (to our knowledge and not including the studies reported in this anthology) regarding empirical applications of the Capability Approach on children, some of which are still unpublished.

As we have argued elsewhere, the capability approach can be operationalised with different methods depending on the purposes of the analysis, the policy implications (e.g. for short- or long-term policies), the choice of focus on either comparability or the local context or the particular project's goals and objectives (Biggeri & Mehrotra, 2010).

In the case of children, it is worth distinguishing between participatory and non-participatory methods according to the different levels of children's involvement (Hart, 1992).[2] In both cases, a starting point of the operationalisation, is often, but not always, represented by the identification of relevant capabilities dimensions of well-being.[3]

M. Biggeri (✉)
Department of Economics, University of Florence, 50127 Florence, Italy
e-mail: mario.biggeri@unifi.it

[1] Most of these are in the domain of education. For example, Sen (e.g., 1992, 1999a, 1999b) underlines the main role education plays in promoting capabilities. Nussbaum (1997, 2006) has developed this facet of capabilities more substantially. Other relevant researches are for example Brighouse (2000); Biggeri (2003); Mehrotra and Biggeri (2002); Saito (2003); Swift (2003); Unterhalter and Brighouse (2003); and more recently the edited volume by Walker and Unterhalter (2007).

[2] See Roger Hart's (1992) definition of participation and O'Kane's (2003) analysis of the concept.

[3] Here "domain" and "dimension" are used interchangeably.

S. Andresen et al. (eds.), *Children and the Good Life*, Children's Well-Being:
Indicators and Research 4, DOI 10.1007/978-90-481-9219-9_6,
© Springer Science+Business Media B.V. 2010

Concerning non-participatory methods (mainly quantitative studies), it is important to know that they usually employ secondary data to analyse children's well-being in functionings and, in few cases, in terms of capabilities. This means that the dimensions considered are constrained by the information contained in the database used (Biggeri & Mehrotra, 2010).

Phipps (2002, p. 493) has used a descriptive approach to measure children's well-being in Canada, Norway and the USA while taking into account some basic functionings. She considered children as people now and not simply as "humans becomings" that is, "their current well-being [that] should count in any assessment of 'social welfare'" (Phipps, 2002, p. 493). When comparing children's well-being in the three countries (USA, Canada and Norway), she selected two key functionings considered more suitable than monetary measures (income or consumption) to illustrate children's condition: physical health and emotional well-being.[4] The results showed the high level of well-being in Norwegian children.

Di Tommaso (2006) has employed a structural equation model defined as MIMIC (Multiple Indicators Multiple Causes approach) to combine different indicators and measure Indian children's well-being.[5] This was considered as a non-observable variable determined by different capacities[6] linked to some functionings[7] that are observable because they are described by specific indicators, and by some exogenous variables that are the external causes of well-being.[8] This research has shown that the external variables with the strongest positive impact on children's well-being are parents' literacy and being a male child.

More recently Addabbo and Di Tommaso (2010) have used the same MIMIC model to measure the capacities of 6–13-year-old Italian children. In particular, they focused on two capabilities: "senses, imagination and thought" and "leisure and play activities".[9] They employed descriptive statistics, an ordered probit model, and a structural equation model to investigate relations between the above-mentioned

---

[4] Physical health was measured by four indicators: weight at birth; number of accidents; presence of limits to a normal physical activity; presence of asthma. Emotional well-being was measured through these indicators: disobedience at school, bullying or cruelty, hyperactivity, lying and being anxious.

[5] The author worked with official statistical data on 3,000 children aged 6–12 years from states in central India.

[6] Capacities were selected from the 10 central capabilities listed by Nussbaum (2000), for example, physical health; senses, imagination and thought; and leisure activities and playing time.

[7] The selected functionings were height and weight related to age, school enrolment and job status (whether the child works inside or outside his/her house or he/she does not work).

[8] External causes were identified as the economic situation of the family, parents' literacy level, child's gender, child's family dimensions, caste and order of birth.

[9] Proxies were constructed to examine attitudes towards education, attendance of arts classes and other types of extracurricular class such as computing and languages. The variables used as indicators of the capability "leisure and play activities" included how often children play in a playground, various types of games and attendance of sports classes. Results were obtained by matching two data sets (using a propensity score method): a Bank of Italy survey on income and wealth for the year 2000, and ISTAT data on families, social subjects and childhood conditions for the year 1998.

indicators, the latent construct for capabilities and a set of covariates. Moreover, they used a new dataset to include family income among the covariates. Like Phipps (2002), Addabbo and Di Tommaso found that "after controlling for parents' education, family income loses importance in determining children's capabilities" (Addabbo & Di Tommaso, 2010). Political, social and, in the Italian case, geographical factors are as important as the economic ones in determining children's well-being.

Paul Anand (2008, unpublished) has focused on very young children. He presents an econometric analysis of a relatively novel element of the GSEOP (German Socio-Economic Panel) dataset containing data on the happiness, capabilities and functionings of children from birth to age 2. A first explorative analysis suggests there is also evidence that functionings or activities help promote child development particularly in cognitive areas: for example singing to or with one's child is particularly related to speech development.

Volkert and Wüst (2009) have performed a quantitative analysis of early childhood agency and capability deprivation using German socioeconomic panel data. Their findings suggest that major non-income indicators, notably household type, number of children in a household, social norms, childcare situation, education of mother and time budget, have major a impact on children's functionings. Among these indicators, they have noticed that social participation and contacts of the children strongly depend on the time parents can spend with each child.

Biggeri, Trani and Mauro (2009) have examined child poverty in its multidimensional character in Afghanistan. They applied the dual cut-off method developed by Alkire and Foster (2008). Child poverty is seen as deprivation of capabilities and related achieved functionings. The case analysed concerns the situation of Afghan children using the survey carried out by Handicap International that took many dimensions of children's well-being into consideration including concepts that are usually missing in standard surveys such as love and care. The data used referred to children aged between 5 and 15 years, with the most deprived ones being aged between 5 and 7 years—especially when non-material aspects such as care and respect were considered.

A recent paper from Roelen and Gassmann (2009) focuses on child poverty with a case study in Vietnam.[10] The paper distils a generic construction process from the analysis of existing child poverty approaches, presenting a tool for clear and transparent development of such approaches. It is then applied to the case of Vietnam, using household survey data in order to illustrate its practical use and develop a Vietnam-specific child poverty approach. Findings suggested that 37% of all children are poor with a large rural/urban divide but no significant differences between boys and girls.

After this brief overview on empirical applications using quantitative methods, we shall now turn to empirical work using participatory methods.

---

[10] This work has focused on children aged 0–16 years.

The first application based on a combination of some focus group discussions with children and a survey was applied in Italy during a congress organised for children (Biggeri, Libanora, Mariani, & Menchini, 2004, Biggeri et al., 2006c, Biggeri, 2007). These are the first studies based on the Capability Approach that try to conceptualise children's capabilities. Since then, the research group at Florence has conducted several studies and field research in India (2005, 2008), Nepal (2008) and Uganda (2005).

The research in Uganda represents the first attempt to use the Capability Approach with children (aged 6–17 years) through a full set of participatory methods (Anich, 2006; Anich, Biggeri, Libanora, & Mariani, 2010; Biggeri & Anich, 2009). The aim of the research was to analyse the deprivation of capabilities among street children in Kampala, Uganda, and the capabilities expansion (or reduction) of former street children participating in rehabilitation projects mainly run by local NGOs. This empirical study explored street children's well-being adopting a different and innovative method of analysis applied to a very large sample. The participatory methods, chosen according to the age of the child, were focus group discussions (FGDs), thematic drawings, mobility mapping, photo essays and life histories obtained through interviews between peers. The results were presented by Biggeri and Anich at a conference on "Childhood and Youth: Choice and Participation" at Sheffield, England (Biggeri et al., 2006b).

Another pioneer study in this area is the research focused on street children in Mauritania carried out by Ballet, Bhukuth, and Radj (2004). This research, based mainly on interviews, revealed that affective capital (defined as the capability of being able to love and be loved by those who care for us) is central to a child's well-being. The authors concluded,

Monetary poverty is often considered as being the main reason of the phenomenon of street children. Yet this hypothesis is not sufficient in the case of Mauritania. There is no question to deny that poverty constitutes a propitious compost of the appearance of the phenomenon but, in any case, it cannot be the direct principal explicative factor. Here it is convenient to talk about affective poverty (p. 3).

Adaptation of participatory methods and new ideas can be quite relevant for this research area. Uyan-Semerci (2006), for instance, in the project "1001 Children, 1001 Wish" in Turkey, tried to operationalise the Capability Approach by examining the letters of children as a way of hearing their voices. She admits that, despite being fundamental, it is a very hard task. She also underlines how a democratic and participatory approach to development studies is a necessity—not only for ethical reasons but also in terms of practical consequences.

One of the most interesting efforts has been made by Comim (2006) in a research project designed to evaluate the impact on children's capabilities of a programme introducing music in some Brazilian primary schools attended mainly by poor children. Comim aimed at challenging the belief according to which the objective measurement of capabilities remains an illusive attempt. The multidimensional, objective and counter-factual nature of capabilities are conceived as pillars in this methodology.

Another interesting example is Kellock and Lawthom's (2010) application of the Capability Approach to investigate children's well-being by using photography. In other words, they used Sen's framework to underpin visual representations of functionings. Current British educational policies and initiatives stipulate that the emotional well-being of primary school children is imperative, and consider that the state of well-being has a strong impact on children's participation and learning at school, as well as their future development. Children aged 8–10 years were invited to explore their own perspectives of well-being using photography as a vehicle for expression. Photography was selected as a research tool because it is a rich visual media for communicating ideas in qualitative studies and it enables children to communicate thoughts and feelings creatively. It is also a useful participative method that does not depend on children's linguistic capabilities.

Children used photography to examine the school environment and the opportunities presented to them and whether they see barriers to achieving their values and aims. Children conceptualised notions of functionings such as being creative, being literate, being physically active and being a friend. These capabilities were further developed with reference to commodities and concepts of freedom within the constraints of the school setting. Children could articulate and recognize visually and simply the complex relationships between the factors that influenced their choices and achieved functioning.

Camfield and Tafere (2010) have focused their attention on the local understandings versus universal prescriptions of what is considered good for children, providing evidence from three Ethiopian communities (*Young Lives*). This study highlights that children and their caregivers each attribute a different meaning to the concept of a "good life" and have different opinions about the means necessary to achieve this well-being. The authors have also tried to figure out how far these views can be understood usefully within Nussbaum's meta-framework of central capabilities.

Furthermore, Camfield's work explores whether the Capability Approach can bridge the gap between shared local understandings of a good life and the universal prescriptions given by global bodies such as UNICEF on what is "good for children". It used qualitative data from group interviews and activities with a sub-sample of children (aged 11–13 years), caregivers and community informants.

Blessone (2008), as reported in her MSc thesis, applied the Capability Approach through some "light" participatory methods in order to assess the impact of the social project "Crescer e Viver" in Rio De Janeiro (Brazil) on the children participating in it by analysing data interviews and focus group discussions.

Serrokh (2010) has investigated the still largely unexplored but prominent topic of microfinance and street children. Could solutions be sought for the future of street children based on working arrangements? Serrokh analyses whether the provision of financial services is an appropriate tool for addressing their needs. Based on participatory research in Bangladesh, the paper highlights the need for a holistic programme in which financial services are provided along with vocational training and social services for street children. Moreover, it argues that savings and credit products need to be designed and delivered in a very specific manner in order to enhance the benefits for these forgotten children.

Horna Padrón and Ballet (2010) concentrate on child agency and identity formation. Their work argues that children are endowed with a capacity for agency even in situations in which they seem to be just victims, and examines this capacity of children in a transitional situation on the streets of Peru. This study has identified children and adolescents who perform various activities on the streets or in the midst of traffic, and explores their impact on their capabilities.

In their research for the Bernard van Leer Foundation, Biggeri and Bonfanti (2009) wanted to understand whether the Capability Approach could serve as an appropriate conceptual framework for young children as well, and whether it could help to plan and evaluate early childhood service provisions. They provided a short introduction to different participatory methods used to evaluate services for children aged 4–7 years and then briefly presented the results of their explorative research in India (2008), whose objective was to let the young children attending a crèche created by Project Why (an Indian NGO) evaluate the services offered to them through participatory methods (Bonfanti, 2009). Although the authors admitted that it is too early to reach any specific conclusions, it is clear that the analysis of children's issues through the capability approach is theoretically very promising for policy design and, when combined with participatory methods, can become a useful tool for practitioners.

Before concluding this section, we wish to point out that the thematic group on Children of the Human Development and Capability Association (HDCA) has organised several seminars, conference panels and international workshops (at which a large part of the papers reported here were presented). The most interesting experience to recall was the international workshop (lasting 1 week) just before the Annual International Conference of the HDCA in New Delhi in 2008. The general aim of this workshop was to improve our understanding of how to apply participatory tools with children within the Capability Approach framework. The workshop had two main explicit objectives: the first was to support the work of Project Why (the NGO kindly hosting us) by exploring its impact on the well-being of the children benefiting from its programmes and, in particular, for the children with special needs. The second objective was to strengthen the work of Project Why by supporting its organisational capacity, including empowerment issues. For the first objective, four different research methods were applied: a photo mapping activity, a card game, an association game and a snake game. For the second objective, a SWOT analysis was applied (for more details, see Biggeri et al., 2008).

In this chapter, I have often used the word "operationalisation" but I have not explained it properly. According to Biggeri and Libanora (2010a), operationalisation is the sequence of activities transforming a theoretical framework into a more or less standardised procedure of practical value for planners, users and beneficiaries (in our case children). According to these two authors, when the Capability Approach is used in project design and social evaluation (including impact assessment), it should focus on what children have reason to value to be able to do and to be regarding the quality of their life. Thus, the subjective, cognitive and reflective position of the children needs always to be linked to the actual constraints and opportunities of the specific domestic, cultural, social, economic and political environment. As Biggeri and Libanora (2010a) point out,

> Agency, knowledge and empowerment have become the common grounds where capability, participatory and process approaches (PA) have increasingly engaged themselves, showing to development scholars and practitioners new ways to deal with quantitative and qualitative data, subjective and objective perceptions, virtual or actual involvement of people in matters that they have reason to value.

The procedure developed by Biggeri and Libanora is based on a structured interview translated into a flexible questionnaire. The flexibility of the questionnaire lies in granting the children themselves the possibility of choosing, in an iterative manner, the relevant dimensions on which the questionnaire is built. In this sense, the questionnaire can also be considered as a "light" participatory tool (Hart, 1992). Indeed, to allow children to participate and to become active actors in the analysis, the procedures have been preceded or accompanied by a set of participatory tools.[11]

The operational procedure is based on four main stages. These constitute the core of the process of thinking, reflecting and participating and should support stakeholders in their attempts to identify the fundamental dimensions of their well-being (see Biggeri et al., 2006c). This is done through an active process of (self-) reflection that helps the child to conceptualise his or her set of capabilities facing at the same time those of all children (as a group) living in the local context, and ask him/her to evaluate the capability expansion or reduction related to a project impact (for the philosophical and experimental foundation and more details, see Biggeri & Libanora, 2010a). In September 2008, in Nepal, we translated this procedure into a game suitable for children aged 6–12 years. This first exploration has been a success in terms of child participation and led to some quite interesting results (Biggeri & Libanora, 2010b).

2 Children and Evolving Capabilities

Although the Capability Approach has been conceived in the context of fully rational human beings with the potential to be part of a social contract, Ballet, Comim, and Biggeri (2010), by holistically embracing the Capability Approach to children,

---

[11] The first procedure has been applied systematically since 2004 by our research group based at Florence University and related to the thematic group on Children's Capabilities of the HDCA while the second procedure has been tested since 2006. We applied this procedure in five studies: at the first Children's World Congress on Child Labour (CWCCL) (Florence, Italy in May 2004) and at the second Children's World Congress on Child Labour and Education (Delhi, India, September 2005) both organized by the Global March Against Child Labour (GMACL) and other grassroots associations (see Biggeri et al., 2006a; Biggeri, 2007), in a study among street children in Uganda (Kampala, March–April 2005, see also next chapter), in India (Delhi, May–September 2008) evaluating the impact of Project Why on disabled children and in Nepal to children and women victims of home violence at the Women Foundation (Kathmandu, September 2008).

do not just affirm that children are the subjects of capabilities but that they may have different capabilities than adults and/or that they can give different degrees of relevance to the same capability.[12,13] In other words, they point out that capabilities should not be viewed within a static (as they usually are) but within a dynamic framework. Furthermore, even more significantly, they underline that we need to recognise that children are social actors endowed with agency and autonomy (according to their maturity) who are able to express (in different ways) their points of view and priorities.[14]

According to Ballet et al. (2010), the Capability Approach and the capability concepts, which, in a certain sense, incorporate the opportunity concept, the capacity concept and the agency concept, evolve over time. The dynamic process of the three components of capabilities can be captured by the notion of *evolving capabilities* (Biggeri, Ballet, & Comim, 2010)[15]:

> The process of evolving capabilities starts from an initial set of achieved functionings of the child. The process of resource conversion is very much affected by how different institutions, norms and cultures constraint or empower them, shaping the formation of a new set of functionings and capabilities that are intertemporally distinct. The child capability set (Opportunity freedom, i.e. the vector of potential valued and achievable functionings, i.e. real) is thus given by the resources/constraints, by his or her limited opportunities and by his or her own abilities. From the capability set the choice will determine the vector of new achieved functionings... The dynamic process is going to be influenced by feedback loops if seen as taking places in sequential periods of time.

The dynamic of the Capability Approach is indeed expressed by the feedback loops that reshape the potential capability set and the capability set of the child. Following Trani, Bakhshi, and Biggeri (2010), the child is conceived at the centre of the development process,[16] interacting and using entitlements available through his or her families, schools, communities and regional/national entities.

Furthermore, as Sen has pointed out—both for children and adults—"while exercising your own choices may be important enough for some types of freedoms, there are a great many other freedoms that depend on the assistance and actions of others and the nature of social arrangements" (Sen, 2007, p. 9). Therefore, the range

---

[12] This sub-section is based partially on the second chapter of the book *Children and the Capability Approach*, edited by Biggeri et al. (2010) and is attributed to the three authors.

[13] In other words, the relevance of capabilities changes for individuals over the course of their lives (Biggeri et al., 2006c, 2010) and, therefore, a child cannot be seen as a scale model of an adult (White, 2002).

[14] Viewing children as social actors is now quite consolidated in the literature and is based on the results of several studies redefining children from passive to active participants who play a dynamic role in their families' lives, communities and societies (see, e.g. Feeny & Boyden, 2004). See also Baraldi (2008).

[15] In the case of children, this concept is quite close in practical terms to the concept of *evolving capacities* presented by Lansdown (2005, p. 3): "the concept of evolving capacities is central to the balance embodied in the convention between recognising children as active agents in their own lives, entitled to be listened to, respected and granted increasing autonomy in the exercise of rights, while also being entitled to protection in accordance with their relative immaturity and youth".

[16] As in new social theory and in ecological theory (see, e.g., Bronfenbrenner, 1995, 1998).

of "possible functionings" for children, their "capability set", may be restricted due to their capacity, or be limited by their social and physical environment. Indeed, the ability to convert resources and commodities into capabilities and functionings[17] depends on individual and social *conversion factors* and often, to an even greater extent, on their parents' or caregivers' capabilities. During early childhood, the "external capabilities" or E-capability given by informal human relationships (Foster & Handy, 2008) may play a central role and be fundamental and instrumental to satisfy the basic capabilities of the child (see Biggeri & Bellanca, 2009). Clearly, when we consider children and, even more in the case of very young children (infants) and severely disabled persons, caregivers' assistance and the E-capability become fundamental.

Ballet et al. (2010) have pointed out how Sen's approach encompasses the idea of the importance of self-determination, especially when it distinguishes between well-being freedom and agency freedom; the latter implying persons' capacity to exercise their own free will (Sen, 1999a). Accepting that there are different degrees of agency brings us to the first important theoretical and practical consideration related to child capabilities (see Biggeri, 2004; Biggeri et al., 2006b). For instance, the fact that the possibility of converting capabilities into functionings also often depends on the decisions of parents, guardians and teachers, implying that the child's conversion factors are subject to further "constraints/resources". However, what we have argued so far does not demonstrate that all children, newborns included, are endowed with agency. Biggeri and Bellanca (2009) have noticed that it may happen that, coordinating each other, several agents carry out a team action, that is, an action in which the individual well-being is pursued and improved thanks to cooperation with other individuals. Therefore, for young children, it may be necessary to shift the focus from the individual agency to the *team agency*, this latter being based on a relationship that is very demanding in terms of mutual confidence. Interestingly, Biggeri and colleagues highlight that all of us experimented with *team agency* when we were children in the relationships with our mothers. Since the time of conception, mother and child become the main actors on a journey, during which the latter will be given life, entitlements and capability and will grow up towards adulthood and full autonomy. Throughout this process, the mother should aim at developing her child's agency. However, in order to reach this objective, she will have to act in terms of *team agency*. Actually, what is at stake is not only the child's present and future well-being, but also his or her mother's quality of life: the more in tune the mother's expression of agency is with that of her child, the higher the level of the mother's quality of life.[18]

---

[17] A functioning is an achievement, whereas a capability is the ability to achieve. Functionings are, in a sense, related more directly to living conditions, because they are different aspects of one's everyday life. Capabilities, in contrast, are notions of freedom in the positive sense: what real opportunities you have regarding the life you may lead (Sen, 1987, p. 36).

[18] Thinking in terms of team agency implies that the relationship babies create with adults, especially with their mothers, has a reciprocal feature and adults' and children's action have to be coordinated. Lengerstee (2007) argues that the mechanism through which adults operationalise children's agency is the "emotional tuning" that discloses the quality of the emotions the adult

3 A First Investigation Using a Focus Group Discussion

Here, we briefly report an explorative retrospective exercise carried out by Biggeri et al. (2006) based on a focus group discussion (FGD) meant to retrospectively disclose some of the above-mentioned characteristics and aspects of children, capabilities and age dynamics.

The FGD was structured into two strongly interrelated parts. The first part was on age, capabilities and the degree of autonomy of choice; the second on the definition of child's activities according to their impact on the child's well-being. Here we concentrate on the first part.

Eight children from South Asian countries (three from Nepal, two from Pakistan and three from India) were invited to participate in the FGD. The group was mixed and composed of boys and girls. All the children (one aged 13 years, one 14, two 15 and four 16) were quite mature, could understand each other, and all understood at least basic-level English (five people assisted in the FGD to help with the translation if needed, i.e. not as participants).[19]

The FGD was implemented in different phases. First, the children agreed on the age and capability categories proposed by the facilitator. Second, they discussed the relevance of each capability according to the age categories and, then, according to the degree of autonomy of choice. They reached a common view and attributed a final assessment of the capability and related autonomy in the process of choice according to the age of the child. The main results of the discussion are reported in Fig. 1.

Although the results of the FGD have to be treated with caution, there are some important observations:

First, the dimensions conceptualised by the children during the survey identified aspects usually neglected in most socioeconomic studies.

Second, the level of relevance of the capability can vary according to age.

Third, the same is observed for the related autonomy issue. Indeed, there is a strong time dynamic in a child's well-being. Agency and autonomy have to be taken into account, and these vary according to the type of dimensions. Actually, each capability included in the list is relevant for all children but the degree of importance of some capabilities changes according to age. For instance, the level of relevance of time autonomy and mobility increases in line with the child's age. Most of the other capabilities move in the opposite direction.

---

thinks the child is feeling. In other words, the adult's action projects towards the baby what the baby has already autonomously produced in a process of self-socialisation.

[19] All except one of the child delegates participating in the FGD were former child labourers who were benefiting from new opportunities as a result of education and vocational training provided by rehabilitation centres or by local civic organisations. Some of these children were still working to pay their education fees. Clearly, they did not need any introduction to the subject of child well-being, and it is important to note that all of them had taken part in meetings on matters related to the issues of the FGD (see Biggeri et al., 2006c).

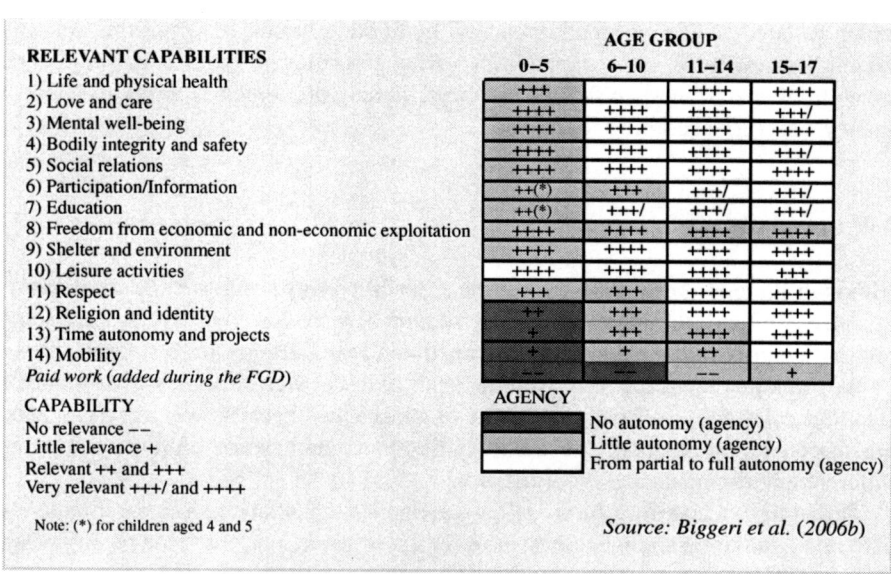

RELEVANT CAPABILITIES	AGE GROUP			
	0–5	6–10	11–14	15–17
1) Life and physical health	+++		++++	++++
2) Love and care	++++	++++	++++	+++/
3) Mental well-being	++++	++++	++++	++++
4) Bodily integrity and safety	++++	++++	++++	+++/
5) Social relations	++++	++++	++++	++++
6) Participation/Information	++(*)	+++	+++/	+++/
7) Education	++(*)	+++/	+++/	+++/
8) Freedom from economic and non-economic exploitation	++++	++++	++++	++++
9) Shelter and environment	++++	++++	++++	++++
10) Leisure activities	++++	++++	++++	+++
11) Respect	+++	+++	++++	++++
12) Religion and identity	++	+++	++++	++++
13) Time autonomy and projects	+	+++	++++	++++
14) Mobility	+	+	++	++++
Paid work (added during the FGD)	--	--	--	+

CAPABILITY

No relevance --
Little relevance +
Relevant ++ and +++
Very relevant +++/ and ++++

AGENCY

No autonomy (agency)
Little autonomy (agency)
From partial to full autonomy (agency)

Note: (*) for children aged 4 and 5   *Source: Biggeri et al. (2006b)*

Fig. 1 FGD results on age, capabilities and agency

Categories used to analyse the level of autonomy were no autonomy, little autonomy and partial or full autonomy. In comparison to capabilities, autonomy of choice increased as children grew older. As expected, the younger the age category, the less degree of freedom in choice the child was expected to have.

It also emerged that for younger children (between 0 and 5 years), some capabilities were considered to be not very relevant (at all, in the case of paid work), and children had no degree of autonomy in the process of choice. This was the case for capabilities such as religion and identity, time autonomy and mobility. According to this retrospective analysis, younger children also had a different degree of autonomy, depending on the capability dimension considered: it is full when leisure activities are concerned, absent in the last three cases (religion and identity, time autonomy and mobility) and low in all other dimensions.

Some remarks made by the children during the FGD indicate the potential usefulness of a further division for the younger age category (0–5). This is in line with the literature that recognises childhood as a period of extraordinary and rapid growth and development, in which cognitive, physical, social, emotional and moral capacities evolve at great speed (Baraldi, 2008; BvLF, 2004; Lansdown, 2005, p. xiii; Rogoff, 1990). For instance, as recalled in a note of Fig. 1, the participants pointed out that some sub-dimensions, such as formal education, only become relevant for children aged 4 and 5.

Another important issue that emerged in the second part of the FGD was the presence of paid work as a capability, but only for older children (aged 15–17 years). This issue was introduced by one girl, but it was not shared by all the other participants. This is a relevant finding, because "paid work" in Nussbaum (2000, 2003) and in Robeyns (2003) is an adult capability. In other words, this confirms not only that the relevance of some capabilities varies according to the age but that some capabilities are adult specific. Furthermore, autonomy, which is an expression of agency, can vary according to the age.

4 Conclusions

Although the possibility of applying the Capability Approach to children is insufficiently explored, the literature review section reveals that there are at least some relevant contributions that already demonstrate the importance of this approach.

We think that the Capability Approach per se is a powerful framework for understanding children's well-being in terms of capabilities because we, as researchers, are forced to think about the complexities that characterise children's lives in different environments and circumstances.

Through the Capability Approach, we are analysing what children are effectively able to do and to be and what they have reason to value, but, for these reasons, "we also should take into account their priorities, strategies and aspirations if we do want use the approach for policy implications" (Ballet et al., 2010).

The evolving capabilities concept and the upgraded framework presented challenge the Capability Approach itself. We conclude that this new, but very promising approach is insufficiently explored and needs to be examined from a multidisciplinary perspective.

Acknowledgements This chapter is strongly rooted in the studies conducted by the research group at the University of Florence since 2003 and its interaction with the members of the thematic group on Children's Capabilities of the Human Development and Capability Association (HDCA) in particular Jeromé Ballet and Flavio Comim to whom we are very thankful. The Florence research group has seen several members Mario Biggeri, Renato Libanora, Nicolò Bellanca, Giovanni Canitano, Stefano Mariani, Vincenzo Mauro, Leonardo Menchini, Simone Bertoli, Rudolf Anich, Sara Bonfanti, Paolo Battistelli, Francesca Marchetta, Aesa Pighini, Enrico Testi and Stefan Zublasing and many other students who have participated in various sessions in Italy and abroad. We are extremely grateful to all of them. Our sincere thanks go to Sabina Alkire, Anou Bakhshi, Parul Bakhshi, Enrica Chiappero Martinetti, David A. Clark, Santosh Mehrotra, Mozaffar Qizilbash, Ingrid Robeyns, Jean-Francois Trani, Alex Frediani, Franco Volpi and Melanie Walker for their useful suggestions during these years. Finally, we wish to thank the University of Bielefeld and in particular Hans Uwe Otto, his research team and Sabine Andresen. The author retains the responsibility for the opinion expressed in the chapter.

References

Addabbo, T., & Di Tommaso, M. L. (2010, forthcoming). Children capabilities and family characteristics in Italy. In M. Biggeri, J. Ballet, & F. Comim (Eds.), *Children and the capability approach* (Chapter 7). Basingstoke: Palgrave Macmillan.

Alkire, S., & Foster, J. E. (2008). *Counting and multidimensional poverty measurement.* (Working Paper No. 7). Oxford, UK: Oxford Poverty and Human Development Initiative (OPHI).

Anand, P. B. (2008). *Homo Faber: The happiness and capabilities of very young children.* Open University, UK: Mimeo, unpublished research.

Anich, R. (2006). Bambini di strada. Indagine sociologica di un recente fenomeno urbano attraverso le parole e le immagini dei bambini di Kampala. Unpublished master's thesis, University of Florence, Italy.

Anich, R., Biggeri, M., Libanora, R., & Mariani, S. (2010, forthcoming). Street children in Kampala and NGOs' action: Understanding capabilities deprivation and expansion. In M. Biggeri, J. Ballet, & F. Comim (Eds.), *Children and the capability approach* (Chapter 5). Basingstoke: Palgrave Macmillan.

Ballet, J., Bhukuth, A., & Radj, K. (2004, September). *Capabilities, affective capital and development application to street children in Mauritania.* Paper presented at the 4th International Conference on the Capability Approach "Enhancing Human Security", Pavia, Italy.

Ballet, J., Comim, F., & Biggeri, M. (2010, forthcoming). Children and the capability approach: Conceptual framework. In M. Biggeri, J. Ballet, & F. Comim (Eds.), *Children and the capability approach* (Chapter 2). Basingstoke: Palgrave Macmillan.

Baraldi, C. (2008). *Bambini e Società.* Rome: Carocci.

Biggeri, M. (2003, September). *Children, child labour and the human capability approach.* Paper presented at the 3rd International Conference on the Capability Approach "From Sustainable Development to Sustainable Freedom", Pavia, Italy.

Biggeri, M. (2004). *Capability approach and child well-being.* Studi e discussioni 141. Florence: Dipartimento di Scienze Economiche, Università degli Studi di Firenze.

Biggeri, M. (2007). Children's valued capabilities. In M. Walker & E. Unterhalter (Eds.), *Amartya Sen's capability approach and social justice in education* (pp. 197–214). New York: Palgrave.

Biggeri, M., & Anich, R. (2009). The deprivation of street children in Kampala: Can the capability approach and participatory methods unlock a new perspective in research and decision making? *Mondes en Développement, 37*(2), 146.

Biggeri, M., Anich, R., Libanora, R., & Mariani, S. (2006a, August). *Street children in Kampala: Understanding capabilities deprivation through participatory methods.* Paper presented at the 5th HDCA annual conference, University of Groningen, Netherlands.

Biggeri, M., Ballet, J., & Comim, F. (Eds.). (2010, forthcoming). *Children and the capability approach.* Basingstoke: Palgrave Macmillan.

Biggeri, M., & Bellanca, N. (2009, September). *Well-being and interpersonal relations of 'weak human beings stakeholders': An enhanced CA framework.* Paper presented at the HDCA annual conference, Lima, Peru.

Biggeri, M., & Bonfanti, S. (2009). *Capability approach and early childhood.* The Hague: Bernard van Leer Foundation.

Biggeri, M., Bonfanti, S., & Conradie, I. (Eds.). (2008, November). *Workshop report: Children's capabilities and project why.* New Delhi, India.

Biggeri, M., & Libanora, R. (2010a, forthcoming). From valuing to evaluating: Tools and procedures to operationalise the capability approach. In M. Biggeri, J. Ballet, & F. Comim (Eds.), *Children and the capability approach* (Chapter 4). Basingstoke: Palgrave Macmillan.

Biggeri, M., & Libanora, R. (2010b, forthcoming). Children's participation in research and decision making.

Biggeri, M., Libanora, R., & Anich, R. (2006b, July). *Children's participation: Can the capability approach unlock a new perspective in research and decision-making?* Paper presented at the international conference "Childhood and Youth: Choice and Participation", University of Sheffield, England.

Biggeri, M., Libanora, R., Mariani, S., & Menchini, L. (2004, September). *Children establishing their capabilities: Preliminary results of the survey during the first children's world congress on child labour.* Paper presented at the 4th International Conference on the Capability Approach "Enhancing Human Security", Pavia, Italy.

Biggeri, M., Libanora, R., Mariani, S., & Menchini, L. (2006c). Children conceptualizing their capabilities: Results of the survey during the first children's world congress on child labour. *Journal of Human Development, 7*(1), 59–83.

Biggeri, M., & Mehrotra, R. (2010, forthcoming). Child poverty as capability deprivation: How to choose dimensions of child well-being and poverty? In M. Biggeri, J. Ballet, & F. Comim (Eds.), *Children and the capability approach* (Chapter 3). Basingstoke: Palgrave Macmillan.

Biggeri, M., Trani, J.-F., & Mauro, V. (2009, June). *The multidimensionality of child poverty: An empirical investigation on children of Afghanistan.* Paper presented at the Workshop on Multidimensional Measures in Six Contexts, Oxford Poverty and Human Development Initiative (OPHI), Oxford, England.

Blessone, I. (2008). *L'approccio delle capacità al concetto di sviluppo e possibili applicazioni empiriche. L'esperienza del circo sociale a Rio de Janeiro.* Unpublished Master's thesis, Università di Torino, Italy.

Bonfanti, S. (2009). *Il capability approach applicato ai bambini: Alcune riflessioni teoriche e il caso di studio di project why a New Delhi.* Unpublished Master's thesis, Università degli studi di Firenze, Italy.

Brighouse, H. (2000). *School choice and social justice.* Oxford: Oxford University Press.

Bronfenbrenner, U. (1995). *Developmental ecology through space and time: A future perspective.* Washington, DC: American Psychological Association.

Bronfenbrenner, U. (1998). The ecology of developmental processes. In U. Bronfenbrenner, P. Morris, W. Damon, & R. M. Lerner (Eds.), *Handbook of child psychology.* Hoboken, NJ: Wiley.

BvLF. (2004). *Early childhood matters.* Review No. 103. The Hague, The Netherlands: Bernard van Leer Foundation.

Camfield, L., & Tafere, Y. (2010, forthcoming). 'Good for children'? Local understandings versus universal prescriptions: Evidence from three Ethiopian communities. In M. Biggeri, J. Ballet, & F. Comim (Eds.), *Children and the capability approach* (Chapter 13). Basingstoke: Palgrave Macmillan.

Comim, F. (2006, August). *Music and the metrics: Evaluating the impact on children's capabilities of social programmes introducing music to primary schools in Brazil.* Paper presented at the 5th HDCA annual conference, University of Groningen, Groningen, The Netherlands.

Di Tommaso, M. L. (2006). *Measuring the well being of children using a capability approach. An application to Indian data.* CHILD Working Papers 05/06. Centre for Household, Income, Labour and Demographic Economics.

Feeny, T., & Boyden, J. (2004). *Acting in adversity: Rethinking the causes, experiences and effects of child poverty in contemporary literature.* (Working Paper No. 116). Oxford, England: Queen Elizabeth House.

Foster, J. E. & Handy, Ch. (2008). External Capabilities. OPHI Working Paper Series No. 08. Oxford: Oxford Poverty ans Human Development Initiative.

Hart, A. R. (1992). *Children's participation: From tokenism to citizenship.* (Essay No. 92/6). Florence, Italy: UNICEF Innocenti Research Centre.

Horna Padrón, M., & Ballet, J. (2010, forthcoming). Child agency and identity: The case of children in a transitional situation in Peru. In M. Biggeri, J. Ballet, & F. Comim (Eds.), *Children and the capability approach* (Chapter 12). Basingstoke: Palgrave Macmillan.

Kellock, A., & Lawthom, R. (2010, forthcoming). Sen's capability approach: Children and well-being explored through the use of photography. In M. Biggeri, J. Ballet, & F. Comim (Eds.), *Children and the capability approach* (Chapter 8). Basingstoke: Palgrave Macmillan.

Lansdown, G. (2005). *The evolving capacities of the child.* Florence: UNICEF Innocenti Research Centre.

Legerstee, M. (2007). *La comprensione sociale precoce.* Milano: Raffaello Cortina (ed. or. 2005).

Mehrotra, S., & Biggeri, M. (2002). *The subterranean child labour force: Subcontracted home based manufacturing in Asia.* (Working Paper No. 96). Florence, Italy: UNICEF Innocenti Research Centre.

Nussbaum, M. (1997). *Cultivating humanity. A classical defence of reform in liberal education.* Cambridge, MA: Harvard University Press.

Nussbaum, M. (2000). *Women and human development: The capabilities approach.* Cambridge: Cambridge University Press.

Nussbaum, M. (2003). Capabilities as fundamental entitlements: Sen and social justice. *Feminist Economics*, *9*(2–3), 33–59.

Nussbaum, M. (2006). *Frontiers of justice: Disability, nationality, species and membership.* London: The Belknap Press.

O' Kane, C. (2003). *Children and young people as citizens: Partners for social change.* London: Save the Children.

Phipps, S. (2002). The well-being of young Canadian children in international perspective: A functioning approach. *Review of Income and Wealth*, *48*, 493–515.

Robeyns, I. (2003). Sen's capability approach and gender inequality: Selecting relevant capabilities. *Feminist Economics*, *9*(2–3), 61–92.

Roelen, K., & Gassmann, F. (2009). *The importance of choice and definition for the measurement of child poverty—the case of Vietnam.* Accessed December 22, 2009, from http://www.springerlink.com/content/j447qm4862572312/

Rogoff, B. (1990). *Apprenticeship in thinking: Cognitive development in social context.* Oxford: Oxford University Press.

Saito, M. (2003). Amartya Sen's capability approach to education: A critical exploration. *Journal of Philosophy of Education*, *37*(1), 17–33.

Sen, A. K. (1987). The standard of living. In G. Hawthorn (Ed.), *The standard of living* (pp. 1–38). Cambridge: Cambridge University Press.

Sen, A. K. (1992). *Inequality re-examined.* Oxford: Oxford University Press.

Sen, A. K. (1999a). *Development as freedom.* Oxford: Oxford University Press.

Sen, A. K. (1999b, November). *Investing in early childhood: Its role in development.* Paper presented at the Conference "Breaking the Poverty Cycle. Investing in Early Childhood", Inter American Development Bank, Washington, DC.

Sen, A. K. (2007). Children and human rights. *Indian Journal of Human Development*, *2*(1), 1–12.

Serrokh, B. (2010, forthcoming). Microfinance, street children and the capability approach: Is microfinance an appropriate tool to address the street children issue? In M. Biggeri, J. Ballet, & F. Comim (Eds.), *Children and the capability approach* (Chapter 11). Basingstoke: Palgrave Macmillan.

Swift, A. (2003). *How not to be a hypocrite: School choice for the morally perplexed.* London: Routledge.

Trani, J.-F., Bakhshi, P., & Biggeri, M. (2010, forthcoming). Re-visiting children's disabilities through the capability approach lens: A framework for analysis and policy implications and an exploration of the Afghanistan case. In M. Biggeri, J. Ballet, & F. Comim (Eds.), *Children and the capability approach* (Chapter 9). Basingstoke: Palgrave Macmillan.

Unterhalter, E., & Brighouse, H. (2003, September). *Distribution of what? How will we know if we have achieved education for all by 2015?* Paper presented at the 3rd International Conference on the Capability Approach "From Sustainable Development to Sustainable Freedom", Pavia, Italy.

Uyan-Semerci, P. (2006, August). *The hard question: How to expand the capabilities of children?* Paper presented at the 5th HDCA annual conference, University of Groningen, Netherlands.

Volkert, J., & Wüst, K. (2009). *Early childhood, agency, and capability deprivation: A quantitative analysis using German socio-economic panel data.* Pforzheim University, Germany: Mimeo, Working Paper.

Walker, M., & Unterhalter, E. (Eds.). (2007). *Amartya Sen's capability approach and social justice in education.* New York: Palgrave.

White, S. C. (2002). Being, becoming and relationship: Conceptual challenges of a child rights approach in development. *Journal of International Development*, *14*(8), 1095–1104.

Subjective Well-Being and Capabilities: Views on the Well-Being of Young Persons

Holger Ziegler

1 The Subjective Well-Being Perspective

The long tradition of the utilitarian philosophy of welfare (cf. Crisp, 1997; Mulgan, 2007) and the new hedonic science of well-being (Huppert, Baylis, & Kaverne, 2005; Layard, 2005) share the suggestion that the value of resources and goods—be they economic, cultural or social—as well as the value of the states and practices of people are not an ontological category. Rather, their value depends upon their relation to the subjective experiences of the persons who benefit or who may be harmed by these goods and states.

This subjective experience might be described in terms of pleasure and pain. If we focus on the overall quality of these subjective experiences, notions such as satisfaction or happiness seem to suggest themselves. And these notions seem to possess high practical relevance. The American pragmatist philosopher William James, for instance, was convinced that the question "how to gain, how to keep, how to recover happiness is in fact for most men at all times the secret motive for all they do" (James, 1902, p. 76). Put differently well-being or happiness is the ultimate objective of human beings (cf. Veenhoven, 1984). Therefore, it is not surprising when authors who are otherwise decisively critical of hedonism and utilitarianism also point to the fact that while inequalities in resources are an important issue, a focus on resources is not sufficient for assessing well-being. Resources are an insufficient information base, because they do not necessarily "tell us what the person will be able to do with those properties" (Sen, 1985, p. 9).

The degree to which individuals have the real and genuine capacity to take advantage of resources and life circumstances points to the in-use value of their opportunities and to the practical significance of opportunities. It does not mean to deny that inequalities matter to people. However, they do not matter so much in terms of the positions, goods and assets which people possess. Rather, inequalities matter in terms of their impact on the lives that people "seek to live and the things,

H. Ziegler (✉)
Faculty of Educational Science, Bielefeld University, 33615 Bielefeld, Germany
e-mail: hziegler@uni-bielefeld.de

S. Andresen et al. (eds.), *Children and the Good Life*, Children's Well-Being: Indicators and Research 4, DOI 10.1007/978-90-481-9219-9_7,
© Springer Science+Business Media B.V. 2010

relationships and practices which they value" (Sayer, 2005, p. 117). Seemingly, the value of resources and opportunities is a practical value assigned by the validation of the acting people themselves. Proponents of utilitarian welfarism and the new hedonic science of well-being comply with this insight. However, they interpret this in a particular way. They argue that people's judgements about their own state (and their own mood) are the primary dimensions for assessing inequality, welfare and the quality of life. Analytically, they embrace the doctrine "agent sovereignty". Their basic argument is that "what is good for each person is entirely determined by that very person's evaluative perspective" (Arneson, 1999, p. 116). This doctrine is typically accompanied by an affirmation of "the principle that, in deciding what is good and what is bad for a given individual, the ultimate criterion can only be his own wants and his own preferences" (Harsanyi, 1982, p. 39). Against this background, subjective life satisfaction—as "the overall appreciation of one's life-as-a-whole" (Veenhoven, 2004)—is considered to be the ultimate criterion for evaluating social conditions of the quality of life. Thus, a measure comes to the forefront that concentrates on an issue that exists only when it is experienced immediately by feeling subjects. Such measures are currently attracting a degree of attention. Supranational institutions, such as the World Health Organization (1993) for instance, have recognised well-being as one of the outcome measures of a health intervention. The idea of subjective well-being is also attracting interest on the political level. The call of scholars to create "National Indicators of Subjective Well-Being and Ill-Being" (Diener, 2006) has been recognised as an important issue of public policy. As the journalist Rana Foroohar points out,

> Policymakers are racing to figure out what makes people happy, and just how they should deliver it... In Britain, a labor economist specializing in happiness—David (Danny) Blanchflower—was recently appointed to the Bank of England advisory board, and the "politics of happiness" will likely figure prominently in next year's elections. Ministers are beginning to consider issues like poverty, health care and transport in relation to "gross national well-being"... the momentum toward a "well-being state" seems unstoppable (Newsweek, April 2007).

In the vein of such a well-being state, Britain's Conservative leader David Cameron proposed a "General Well-Being" index (but Labour has also bought into the politics of happiness). Likewise, the French President Nicolas Sarkozy has recently suggested a happiness index to be added in terms of a further GDP criterion. It can hardly be denied that the idea of happiness as a central objective of public policy is being taken seriously (cf. Duncan, 2008; Ng & Ho, 2006).

Against this background, the new hedonic science of well-being is evolving into an important politically applied science. This is all the more the case as there is evidence that there are valid ways to investigate and measure subjective life satisfaction. One view in the literature reveals that the quest to assess individuals' evaluations of their life satisfaction on the fundament of their cognitive assessment of their overall life quality has been adopted in sociological and psychological research on social indicators. The basic idea of these studies seems to follow Angus Campbell's suggestion that "ultimately the quality of life must be in the eye of the beholder [... and therefore] it is there is there that we seek ways to evaluate it" (Campbell, 1972, p. 442).

Research on subjective well-being is centred not only in the social sciences but also and all the more in economics. In economics, happiness research is suggested to be "a new approach to measuring utility in the context of cost-benefit analysis" (Frey & Stutzer, 2005, p. 208), and the increasing arsenal of psychometric measures of well-being is credited "to contain substantial amounts of valid variance" (Diener, 1984, p. 551).

On the level of assessing inequalities in well-being, economic studies typically follow the tradition of utilitarianism. Most basically utilitarianism—in the tradition of Jeremy Bentham and John Stuart Mill—suggests that the preferable state of a distribution of valued goods or, more precisely, of utility is characterised by the greatest good for the greatest number of people. As utility is defined as well-being or happiness, this idea is tantamount to the so-called "greatest happiness principle". Subsequently, the quest is to "maximize aggregate happiness as a social welfare function" (Frey & Stutzer, 2007). Accordingly, a state (of distribution) is collectively preferred, when it provides the most positive total of happiness. If $u_p(a)$ respectively $u_p(b)$ is the amount of happiness of person p experiencing state a respectively state b, then state a is preferred to state b whenever

$$\sum_{p=1}^{n} u_p(a) > \sum_{p=1}^{n} u_p(b)$$

Such a summation is only meaningful when we can reasonably assume happiness to be more than an elusive concept that we cannot measure (cf. Veenhoven, 2004) but rather a relatively global and stable attribute (cf. Pavot, Diener, Colvin, & Sandvik, 1991) that is cardinally measurable and interpersonally comparable. Basically, this seems to be the case (cf. Layard, 2005; Ng, 1996), so that happiness might be included in sociological, psychological and economic models.

Happiness seems to be measurable in a comparatively simple way on the basis of psychometric survey measures. Interestingly, results from brain research also confirm that responses to questions about subjective well-being correspond to neurological activities in the regions of the brain assumed to be responsible for the experience of happiness (cf. Kahneman & Krueger, 2006; Urry et al., 2004).

One of the scales considered to be a valid and reliable measure of life satisfaction is the Satisfaction with Life Scale (SWLS) (cf. Diener, Emmons, Larsen, & Griffin, 1985). The SWLS is a widely accepted and one of the most widely used tools for measuring well-being.

In a survey study with 141 boys and girls aged 13–17 years in the German city of Bielefeld, we applied the SWLS as a measure of subjective well-being. Interestingly well-being was very much related to aspects of affiliation and relations. In a linear regression, about 30% of the variance in the subjective well-being of these young persons was explained by the three factors "Emotional support" (cf. Schulz & Schwarzer, 2003), "Feelings of social exclusion" (Bude & Lantermann, 2006) and the quality of "Relations to parents".[1] The most significant factor, "Emotional support," was highly correlated in turn with "Having good and reliable friends" ($r = 0.572$). Of course, other more individual aspects such as self-esteem (measured by means of the Rosenberg Self-Esteem Scale, cf. Rosenberg, 1965) and self-efficacy (measured by means of the Generalised Self-Efficacy Scale) are also highly related to subjective well-being. However, when they are added to the regression model, these factors prove to neither relevantly improve the explained variance of the model, nor to be significant coefficients influencing subjective well-being.

This result is consistent with a growing body of evidence suggesting a strong relation between different aspects and dimensions of "social capital" and "subjective well-being" (cf. Gundelach & Kreiner, 2004; Helliwell, 2006; Helliwell & Putnam, 2005; Winkelmann, 2009). More importantly, it confirms studies on children like the World Vision study on Children 2007 indicating that family and friends are decisively relevant background variables for the well-being of children aged 8–11 years (Andresen & Hurrelmann, 2007). In a German study on socially disadvantaged children, Sabine Andresen and Susann Fegter (2009) have also pointed out that almost all children mention that having good caring relationships with parents and having nice and reliable friends are among the most important dimensions in what constitutes a good life for children. Obviously, when we talk about the well-being of children, we have to take into account the quality of their relations and affiliations (cf. Bucher, 2001).

In our study in Bielefeld, the type of school the young persons were attending had virtually no impact on their subjective life satisfaction. And there was also no correlation between their well-being and the educational qualifications of their parents. This is interesting, because, in Germany, educational qualifications are an exceptionally robust indicator of social class (cf. Geißler, 2002). These results comply with the insight that socio-demographic variables do not explain much of the variance in the happiness of children (cf. Bucher, 2001). This is also confirmed by the latest large-scale Youth Survey conducted by the German Youth Institute (GYI) in which 2,154 young persons aged 12–15 years were interviewed. This survey also suggested that not only major life events, such as the breakdown of an important friendship, the divorce of one's parents, but also the death of important friends or even the death of one's parents are—in the long run—not correlated with the happiness of children.

However, what seems to be most significant is that the data of the GYI Youth Survey indicate that 97.9% of 12–15-year-old Germans are very or rather happy with their overall life. The same is true for 92.9% of those aged 16–27. This is interesting, because studies using more "objective" measures of well-being come to decisively different conclusions about the quality of life of young people in Germany

---

[1] Relations to parents is an outcome of mean component analyses with the items "I have great respect for my parents," "My parents respect my opinion," "I enjoy spending time with my parents," "Whenever I have problems, I can turn to my parents," "My parents are great" and, reverse coded, "I have trouble with my parents". Factor loadings are high (between 0.702 and 0.826), and the factor captures 54% of the variance and has an internal consistency of $\alpha = 0.84$.

(cf. Bertram, 2006; UNICEF, 2007). The results of the GYI Survey have been replicated in a range of other studies. In our Bielefeld study, 89% of the teenagers were very or rather satisfied with their lives measured in terms of the SWLS. Even in the study of Andresen and Fegter (2009), clearly more than 80% of the young children considered themselves to be happy despite being exposed to multiple social and economic disadvantages. Put differently, when the quality of life of young persons in Germany is defined in terms of their subjective well-being, the world in Germany seems to be fine, even though there are undeniable and significant inequalities in terms of the economic, social and cultural resources these young persons possess.

Even more disturbing might be the fact that, as Mark Kelman (2005) points out, a range of studies suggest,

> that a variety of social programs that reduced social expectations among the disadvantaged might be hedonically beneficial as well. The key empirical findings here are that increasing the social isolation of subordinated groups often seems to make them happier by leading individuals to compare themselves to a narrower, less prosperous cohort in evaluating their circumstances. Thus, women reported themselves to be more satisfied with their incomes when they did not have much chance of getting traditionally male jobs at male pay. Black children in segregated schools have substantially higher self-esteem than blacks in integrated settings and than white children (without regard to school setting), while high-status blacks—who interact with more whites and expect to have lives more like theirs—were reported by some researchers to have low and falling rates of happiness (p. 400).

Kelman (2005, p. 401) goes on to summarise that it seems to be clear "that as long as individuals do as well as those around them who form a salient, recognized social group, they feel pretty satisfied". This implies, however, that in terms of its impact on subjective well-being, a "stable and unquestioned hierarchy. . . seems to dominate fluidity (which leads largely to higher, disappointed expectations, or to self-blame for bad outcomes)" (ibid.). Also on the level of policies of well-being, these assumptions of the protagonists of subjective well-being, that "quality of life must be in the eye of the beholder" (Campbell, 1972) have quite radical consequences: Taken seriously, this perspective on well-being implies to be "indifferent between policies that increase people's opportunities and those that dampen their expectations if the two policies have identical impacts on subjective well-being" (Kelman, 2005, p. 401).

A number of studies have pointed to the problem of "adaptive preferences" that is, "preferences that have adjusted to their second-class status" (Nussbaum, 2003, p. 33) or to circumstances that may be "objectively" unfavourable. Adaptive preferences point to the fact that while "people's own assessment of their degree of satisfaction [. . .] is partly determined by their level of aspiration" (Erikson, 1993, p. 77), it is known that, by and by, people in distressed situations become accustomed to and tend to conform to unfavourable circumstances. As David Swartz (2000) puts it, the process of adaptive internalisation

> tends to shape individual action so that existing opportunity structures are perpetuated. Chances of success or failure are internalized and then transformed into individual aspirations or expectations; these are then in turn externalized in action that tends to reproduce the objective structure of life chances (p. 103).

Such a "quiet acceptance of deprivation and bad fate affects the scale of dis-satisfaction generated" (Sen, 1984, p. 309). Referring to processes of adapting preferences, some commentators go so far as to suggest that "measuring how sat-isfied people are is to a large extent equivalent to measuring how well they have adapted to their present" (Erikson, 1993, p. 77). As a "utilitarian calculus gives sanc-tity to that distortion" (Sen, 1984, p. 309), happiness and life satisfaction as proxies for utility are rather "inadequate as a basis of social choice" (Nussbaum, 2000, p. 139) and subsequently a misleading fundament for social policy. As Bruckner (2009) puts it,

> The trouble comes when social policy is driven by people's actual preferences. If what people in oppressed circumstances want is conditioned by their presently-feasible options, no social action would seem to be called for to improve the lot of such oppressed people who do not express dissatisfaction with their circumstances (p. 311).

Even more disturbing might be the fact that policies and ideologies that obscure injustice, oppression and inequality may well be conducive to happiness, whereas consciousness-raising may induce dissatisfaction. In a survey with single mothers on welfare, for instance, it became obvious that the personal belief in a just world (cf. Lerner, 1980), even when facing considerable social distress, correlates highly with SWLS ($r = 0.327$).

The problems with subjective approaches to assessing well-being are obvious. Nevertheless, it is still convincing that inequalities matter most in terms of their impact on the lives that people—including young people—"seek to live and the things, relationships and practices which they value" (Sayer, 2005, p. 117). Against this background, we have to accept that an assessment of "objective" resources is not a sufficient information base for well-being. Yet this insight of Andrew Sayer does not necessarily make a point in favour of subjective approaches to well-being. Rather, he stresses the significance of use value and internal goods. The idea is therefore to focus not just on cash or in-kind resources, but on a whole configura-tion of resources, and individual and social factors that allow individuals to convert resources into valuable states and activities (cf. Bonvin, 2009). This configuration could be regarded as a person's capability set. Following this perspective, Sayer argues that the inequalities that matter most "effect what Amartya Sen calls... [people's] 'capabilities' to engage in ways of life they have reason to value". My argument is that a focus on such capabilities is a more appropriate way to assess the well-being and quality of life of young people than assessing their happiness or their material resources or a combination of both.

2 The Capabilities Perspective

The Capabilities Approach (CA) is associated with the names of the Indian economist Amartya Sen and the American philosopher Martha Craven Nussbaum. Initially, it was a philosophical approach attempting to reconcile the competing demands associated with the fundamental conceptions of equality, recognition and liberty. The central issue of the CA is the issue of a good life, respectively, a successful conduct of life. As a result, the CA is concerned with the cultivation, maximization and just distribution of the (real) freedom and the well-being of persons.[2] When addressing this, the CA focuses on the arrangement of the different behaviours and various lifestyles individuals have at their disposal and, as a result, the question of their positive freedom to decide for a life they have reason to value. As Martha Nussbaum (2000) summarises,

> We ask not only about the person's satisfaction with what she does, but about what she does, and what she is in a position to do (what her opportunities and liberties are). And we ask not just about the resources that are sitting around, but about how those do or do not go to work, enabling [this person] to function in a fully human way (p. 71).

In their argumentation for the CA, both Sen and Nussbaum basically follow an Aristotelian ethic that considers a "virtuous character" to be a fundamental prerequisite for living such a good life. Such a focus on a theory of virtue is attractive for a kind of research that focuses on the complexity of living environments and lifestyles and agents "with a concrete history, identity and affective-emotional constitution" (Benhabib, 1989, p. 460), as well as on the issue of culture, that is, "attitudes, mindsets and symbolically articulated conceptions of life" (Brumlik, 2007, p. 82). Following the Aristotelian tradition, the CA goes beyond rules, standards, principles and rational decision making and takes into account desires, tendencies, feelings, attitudes, perspectives on past experiences, systems of meaning and of symbols as well as aesthetic motivations behind actions, referring to the fact that a good life is not only an individual project, but at all times also a social one.

The reference to the Aristotelian teachings of virtue at the same time connects the CA to a tradition that assumes that a good life can be accomplished when people live their lives according to their specific, idiosyncratic dispositions. Yet this proposition alone might be reason enough to remain sceptical towards the CA. Such a conceptualisation of a good life claims at least a basic understanding of what a "true human life" is, in order to derive from this understanding an objective definition of what is good and what a well-managed and fulfilled life is. Every attempt to substantially define a good, successful or happy life in this way raises suspicions of metaphysical-teleological essentialism. Particularly when the good life in established interpretations of the Aristotelian model of goodness is considered with

---

[2]This concern has strong similarities with the notion of *Bildung*, a key concept in continental European (and, in particular, German-speaking) traditions of educational theory. If we eclipse the fact that the notion of *Bildung* also legitimised the ideals of an elitist educational ideology of the bourgeoisie, *Bildung* implies a practice that transcends a mere acquisition of knowledge (cf. Bleicher, 2006). Josef Bleicher has figured out that "*Bildung* points to a way of integrating knowledge and expertise with moral and aesthetic concerns. On the basis of a successful integration of thinking, willing and feeling, it enables sound judgement, indicated by a developed awareness of what is appropriate. . . It entails openness to difference and a willingness to self-correct. *Bildung*, in the classic sense, thus also contains a projective anticipation of the 'good life', of human freedom enacted with responsibility for self and others in the open-ended project of self-creation" (Bleicher, 2006, p. 365).

regard to the fulfilment of essential dispositions and abilities, instead of the self-realisation of individual originality and uniqueness, "become-who-you-are" theories based upon this view (cf. Horn, 2006) may lead to reactionary forms of criticism of modernisation. This might be found, for instance, in traditionalist argumentations for natural justice as well as in neoconservative versions of communitarianism. With reference to this tradition, educational and policy attempts may legitimise authoritative decisions about "what people were to consider as their happiness" (Seel, 1998, p. 113), and decree what was good for all on the basis of the lifestyles of some third parties. Such an approach would be authoritarian, and it would diametrically oppose enlightened and emancipatory conceptions: A generally mandatory, detailed definition of what is good amounts to the questioning of basic liberal and value-pluralistic premises. To decree a material definition of what is good would not only mean an anti-pluralistic arrogance tending towards totalitarianism and an "unbearable paternalism" (Habermas, 1996, p. 42), but could also hardly be justified by any logic of argumentation. For, as Habermas (1996) points out,

> before engaging in any moral deliberation, those involved would have to know what is equally good for all. However, no one can simply assess from an observing perspective what any person should consider to be good. The reference to 'any' person implies an abstraction that asks too much of philosophers even [as well as policy makers, teachers, or social workers] (p. 44).

Approaches that claim to be able to decide "objectively" about conceptions that have always been morally and politically disputed—such as that of what is good—may lead to ideologies hardly reconcilable with modern concepts of autonomy. The CA is *not* one of those ideologies—even though it is based on a "thick vague conception of the human good" (Nussbaum, 1995, p. 456) and is concerned with the creation and maintenance of social circumstances that allow individuals to live successful lives.

According to Nussbaum (1999), the essential public function is to

> Make available to each and every citizen the material, institutional, and educational circumstances in which good human functioning may be chosen; to move each and every one of them across a threshold of capability into circumstances in which they may choose to live and function well (p. 24).

However, the CA neither aims to impose an understanding of what is good on the agents, nor to constrain their freedom of doing and being with respect to that aim, nor does it support (the government) "to force people into excellence" (Hurka, 1993, p. 147). On the contrary, the CA represents one of the modern, liberal approaches to a definition of what is good that ask "what it can mean for a person to strive for well-being and happiness and to avoid suffering, hardships and misery (as far as possible),... [not from a general view from nowhere] but from the hypothetic perspective of any individual" (Seel, 1998, p. 114).

Against this theoretical background, the CA represents an approach concerned with the scope of self-determination and autonomy to render a good life possible. The CA takes this focus on the scope of opportunities and the freedom of people to live their own lives seriously and in a systematic fashion, by differentiating between functionings and chances of realisation, respectively capabilities.

Functionings refer to the question whether people actually are or do something specific. In contrast to this, the perspective of capabilities is directed towards the *objective set* of opportunities to realise *different combinations* of certain qualities and functionings. Considering the chances of realisation, what matters is the *real, practical freedom* of people to *decide* for or against the realisation of certain functions and lifestyles, that is, being able to develop and to realise one's own conception of a good life (cf. Sen, 1992, 1999). This objective real freedom and the suitable institutional conditions enabling and facilitating this freedom are considered to be the good to be advanced. This means the CA is less concerned with establishing a coercion and discipline towards the "good", but rather with a definition of the basic opportunities and capacities as well as their implementation to which people are entitled and that can be understood as the basis of the pursuit and realisation of various plans or designs of a good life (cf. Nussbaum, 2000).

Therefore, on the one hand, research on the basis of the CA is about whether people have access to what they reasonably aspire to be and to do. On the other hand, and most importantly, capabilities-oriented research on well-being is also about whether people have the real and genuine freedom to choose among such options. At the centre of concern is therefore "the extent of freedom (negative and positive) people have to achieve doings and beings that they (have reason to) value" (Wolff & de-Shalit, 2007, p. 37). In terms of inequality therefore, the fundamental metric is "the capability each has to enjoy valuable activities and states of being" (Alkire, 2002, p. 4).

From the viewpoint of the CA, the important factors are the range and quality of the spectrum as well as the number of those opportunities and capacities of people to be able to realise doings and beings important to their own concept of a good life that can be effectively realised and differentiated. This is what has to be measured and reconstructed *empirically*.

Therefore the CA assigns a specific task to research on the well-being of (particularly young) persons: to develop a relational perspective that makes it possible to relate the materially, culturally and political-institutionally structured domain of social opportunities to young people's domain of individual agency and the ability to self-actualise. Together, these possibilities and capacities determine the objective chances of well-being in the sense of a good life. The good life, to be defined in this way, is the central target term and in-use value of a socially reflexive reorientation of research on children and youth.

References

Alkire, S. (2002). *Valuing freedoms. Sen's capability approach and poverty reduction.* Oxford: Oxford University Press.

Andresen, S., & Fegter, S. (2009). *Spielräume sozial benachteiligter Kinder.* Leverkusen: Bayer Vital GmbH.

Andresen, S., & Hurrelmann, K. (2007). *World Vision Deutschland: Kinder in Deutschland 2007. 1. World Vision Kinderstudie.* Frankfurt a. M.: Fischer.

Arneson, R. J. (1999). Human flourishing versus desire satisfaction. *Social Philosophy and Policy, 16*(1), 113–143.

Benhabib, S. (1989). Der verallgemeinerte und der konkrete Andere. Ansätze zu einer feministischen Moraltheorie. In E. List & H. Studer (Eds.), *Denkverhältnisse* (pp. 454–487). Frankfurt a. M.: Suhrkamp.

Bertram, H. (2006). *Zur Lage der Kinder in Deutschland: Politik für Kinder als Zukunftsgestaltung.* (Innocenti Working Paper No. 2006-02). Florence, Italy: UNICEF Innocenti Research Centre.

Bleicher, J. (2006). Bildung. *Theory, Culture & Society, 23,* 364–365.

Bonvin, J.-M. (2009). Der Capability Ansatz und sein Beitrag für die Analyse gegenwärtiger Sozialpolitik. *Soziale Passagen, 1,* 8–22.

Bruckner, D. (2009). In defense of adaptive preferences. *Philosophical Studies, 142*(3), 307–324.

Brumlik, M. (2007). Soll ich je zum Augenblicke sagen. . . Das Glück: Beseligender Augenblick oder erfülltes Leben? In F. Kessl (Ed.), *Erziehung zur Armut? Soziale Arbeit und die,neue Unterschicht'* (pp. 81–96). Wiesbaden: VS-Verlag.

Bucher, A. (2001). *Was Kinder glücklich macht. Historische, psychologische und empirische Annäherungen an Kindheitsglück.* Weinheim: Juventa.

Bude, H., & Lantermann, E.-D. (2006). Soziale Exklusion und Exklusionsempfinden. *Kölner Zeitschrift für Soziologie und Sozialpsychologie, 58*(2), 233–252.

Campbell, A. (1972). Aspiration, satisfaction and fulfillment. In A. Campbell & P. Converse (Eds.), *The human meaning of social change* (pp. 441–466). New York: Russell Sage Foundation.

Crisp, R. (1997). *Routledge philosophy guidebook to Mill on utilitarianism.* London: Routledge.

Diener, E. (1984). Subjective well-being. *Psychological Bulletin, 95*(3), 542–575.

Diener, E. (2006). Guidelines for national indicators of subjective well-being and ill-being. *Journal of Happiness Studies, 7,* 397–404.

Diener, E., Emmons, R., Larsen, R., & Griffin, S. (1985). The satisfaction with life scale. *Journal of Personality Assessment, 49,* 71–75.

Duncan, G. (2008). Should happiness-maximization be the goal of government? *Journal of Happiness Studies,* doi: 10.1007/s10902-008-9129-y.

Erikson, R. (1993). Descriptions of inequality: The Swedish approach to welfare. In M. Nussbaum & A. Sen (Eds.), *The quality of life* (pp. 67–83). Oxford: Clarendon Press.

Frey, B., & Stutzer, A. (2005). Happiness research: State and prospects. *Review of Social Economy, 62*(2), 207–228.

Frey, B., & Stutzer, A. (2007). *Should national happiness be maximized?* (Working Paper 306). Zurich, Switzerland: University of Zurich, Institute for Empirical Research in Economics.

Geißler, R. (2002). *Die Sozialstruktur Deutschlands. Die gesellschaftliche Entwicklung vor und nach der Vereinigung.* Wiesbaden: VS-Verlag.

Gundelach, P., & Kreiner, S. (2004). Happiness and life satisfaction in advanced European countries. *Cross-Cultural Research, 38,* 359–386.

Habermas, J. (1996). Eine genealogische Betrachtung zum kognitiven Gehalt der Moral. In J. Habermas (Ed.), *Die Einbeziehung des Anderen. Studien zur politischen Theorie* (pp. 11–64). Frankfurt a. M.: Suhrkamp.

Harsanyi, J. (1982). Morality and the theory of rational behavior. In A. Sen & B. Williams (Eds.), *Utilitarianism and beyond* (pp. 39–62). Cambridge: Cambridge University Press.

Helliwell, J. (2006). Well-being, social capital, and public sector – What's new? *The Economic Journal, 116*(510), 34–45.

Helliwell, J., & Putnam, R. (2005). The social context of well-being. In F. Huppert, N. Baylis, & B. Kaverne (Eds.), *The science of well-being* (pp. 435–459). Oxford: Oxford University Press.

Horn, C. (2006). Glück/Wohlergehen. In M. Düwell, C. Hübenthal, & M. Werner (Eds.), *Handbuch ethik* (pp. 381–387). Stuttgart/Weimar: Metzler.

Huppert, F. A., Baylis, N., & Kaverne, B. (Eds.). (2005). *The science of well-being.* Oxford: Oxford University Press.

Hurka, T. (1993). *Perfectionism.* Oxford: Oxford University Press.

James, W. (1902). *Varieties of religious experience.* New York: Barnes & Noble.

Kahneman, D., & Krueger, A. (2006). Developments in the measurement of subjective well-being. *Journal of Economic Perspectives, 20*(1), 3–24.

Kelman, M. (2005). Hedonic psychology and the ambiguities of welfare. *Philosophy and Public Affairs*, *33*(4), 391–412.

Layard, R. (2005). *Happiness*: *Lessons from a new science*. New York/London: Penguin.

Lerner, M. (1980). *The belief in a just world*. New York: Plenum Press.

Mulgan, T. (2007). *Understanding utilitarianism*. Stocksfield: Acumen.

Ng, Y.-K. (1996). Happiness surveys: Some comparability issues and an exploratory survey based on just perceivable increments. *Social Indicators Research*, *38*(1), 1–27.

Ng, Y.-K., & Ho, L. S. (2006). Introduction: Happiness as the only ultimate objective of public policy. In Y.-K. Ng & L. S. Ho (Eds.), *Happiness and public policy*: *Theory, case studies and implications* (pp. 1–16). Houndmills: Palgrave Macmillan.

Nussbaum, M. (1995). Human functioning and social justice: In defence of Aristotelian essentialism. In D. Tallack (Ed.), *Critical theory*: *A reader* (pp. 449–472). New York: Harvester Wheatsheaf.

Nussbaum, M. (1999). *Gerechtigkeit oder Das gute Leben*. Frankfurt a. M.: Suhrkamp.

Nussbaum, M. (2000). *Women and human development*: *The capabilities approach*. Cambridge: Cambridge University Press.

Nussbaum, M., (2003) Capabilities as fundamental entitlements: Sen and social justice. *Feminist Economics*, 2(3), 33–60.

Pavot, W., Diener, E., Colvin, C. R., & Sandvik, E. (1991). Further validation of the satisfaction with life scale: Evidence for the cross-method convergence of well-being measures. *Journal of Personality Assessment*, *57*(1), 149–161.

Rosenberg, M. (1965). *Society and the adolescent self-image*. Princeton, NJ: Princeton University Press.

Sayer, A. (2005). *The moral significance of class*. Cambridge: Cambridge University Press.

Schulz, U., & Schwarzer, R. (2003). Soziale Unterstützung bei der Krankheitsbewältigung. Die Berliner Social Support Skalen (BSSS). *Diagnostica*, *49*, 73–82.

Schwarzer, R., & Jerusalem, M. (1995). Generalized self-efficacy scale. In J. Weinman, S. Wright, & M. Johnston (Eds.), *Measures in health psychology*: *A user's portfolio. Causal and control beliefs* (pp. 35–37). Windsor: NFER Nelson.

Seel, M. (1998). Wege einer Philosophie des Glücks. In J. Schummer (Ed.), *Glück und Ethik* (pp. 109–123). Würzburg: Königshausen & Neumann.

Sen, A. (1984). *Resources, values and development*. Oxford: Blackwell.

Sen, A. (1985). *Commodities and capabilities* (Prof. Dr. P. Hennipman Lectures in Economics Vol. 7). Amsterdam: Elsevier Science.

Sen, A. (1992). *Inequality re-examined*. Oxford: Oxford University Press.

Sen, A. (1999). *Development as freedom*. Oxford: Oxford University Press.

Swartz, D. (2000). *Culture and power*: *The sociology of Pierre Bourdieu*. Chicago: University of Chicago Press.

UNICEF. (2007). *An overview of child well-being in rich countries*. Florence: UNICEF Innocenti Research Centre.

Urry, H., Nitschke, J. B., Dolski, I., Jackson, D. C., Dalton, K. M., Mueller, C. J., et al. (2004). Making a life worth living: Neural correlates of well-being. *Psychological Science*, *15*, 367–372.

Veenhoven, R. (1984). *Conditions of happiness*. Dordrecht: Reidel.

Veenhoven, R. (2004). Happiness as an aim in public policy: The greatest happiness principle. In P. Linley & S. Joseph (Eds.), *Positive psychology in practice* (pp. 658–678). New York: Wiley.

Winkelmann, R. (2009). Unemployment, social capital, and subjective well-being. *Journal of Happiness Studies*, *10*(4), 421–430.

Wolff, J., & de-Shalit, A. (2007). *Disadvantage*. Oxford: Oxford University Press.

World Health Organization. (1993). *WHOQOL study protocol*. Geneva: Author.

Language Education—For the "Good Life"?

Isabell Diehm and Veronika Magyar-Haas

1 Introduction

Since the first Programme for International Student Assessment (PISA) findings were announced in the year 2001 with the resulting "PISA shock" due to Germany's poor performance, early language education has generally been considered a must for elementary education practice in the German context. Since then, expectations and demands have focused on supporting children's language development more purposefully than before in order to secure later success at school. This should ensure sufficiently developed language skills at school entrance to make it easy for children to take part in lessons during their first years of primary school. This is particularly meant for children whose first or family language is not German due to a migration background (see Apeltauer, 2007). In so far, these are primarily goal-oriented, instrumental considerations connecting early language support with later reading skills.

Accordingly, the educational curricula at kindergartens and day nurseries in the individual German federal states, though only in existence for a few years, place great emphasis on the importance of language support, often understood as *language education* (*sprachliche Bildung*) at Kindergarten.[1] Additionally, concrete educational policy guidelines have now resulted in a general introduction of language tests before starting school and a variety of support activities in the field of elementary education. Different methods of evaluating language skills, mostly in the form of measurement or screening tools (see Lütje-Klose, 2007), as well as a wide range of language trainings and programmes have been developed and are now to be found in all federal states. However, their implementation is completely homogeneous—differing in every federal state, every municipality and every institution. Likewise, there have been hardly any evaluations of their effectiveness and intervention effects up to now.

I. Diehm (✉)
Faculty of Educational Science, Bielefeld University, 33615 Bielefeld, Germany
e-mail: isabell.diehm@uni-bielefeld.de

[1] See the different curricula of the individual federal states.

S. Andresen et al. (eds.), *Children and the Good Life*, Children's Well-Being:
Indicators and Research 4, DOI 10.1007/978-90-481-9219-9_8,
© Springer Science+Business Media B.V. 2010

In this context, it is still unclear to what extent the implemented methods of diagnosis and intervention approaches can be viewed as individual or group-related measures. Indeed, these stages mostly claim to be individual language interventions, oriented towards the needs of individual children.[2] In most cases, support is provided—like training courses—in small groups, separated or isolated from everyday play and the action contexts of kindergartens.

Apart from the ubiquitously used term *language intervention*, the relevant literature also uses the term *language education*. Hardly any distinction is drawn between the two terms, and their theoretical embedment also remains vague.

Against the background of this nationally coded sketch of the problem, this chapter draws on Nussbaum's (2000, 2005) Capabilities Approach to first theoretically discuss the relevance of language and literacy for a "*good life*" and the successful and favourable growing up of children—an approach that has yet to be taken into consideration in the German debate on language, language education and language support. The next section sheds more light on the concept of (early) language education from the point of view of the Capabilities Approach and what it substantially has to offer. This will be followed by insights from a pilot study using the method of participant observation during everyday activities at kindergartens to find out how language is lived and promoted there. This observation study was not interested in the language skills of individual children but in the value of language and literacy in everyday life. The next section examines the existing institutional resources that provide what is called the educational arrangement. Finally, conclusions are sketched on which basic capabilities are necessary to make social (and political) participation possible.

2 The Relevance of Language and Literacy in the Context of the Capabilities Approach

For more than two decades, the philosopher Martha Nussbaum (1988, 1990, 1999) has been pursuing the question of a "good life". Based on her experiences as a research advisor at the World Institute for Development Economics Research in Helsinki since 1986 as well as on discussions with women's development projects in India, she sketched a universalistic, feminist political philosophy rooted in Aristotle.[3] She claims to introduce new topics into her agenda, such as "hunger

---

[2]See the FÖRMIG (*Förderung von Kindern mit Migrationshintergrund* [support for children with a migration background]) model programme organized by the Institut für Internationale und Interkulturell Vergleichende Erziehungswissenschaft of the University of Hamburg with the support of the Bund-Länder-Kommission (BLK). This is currently one of the biggest and most extensive language intervention projects.

[3]Nussbaum (1990, p. 203) emphasises that the task of political planning in Aristotle was "to make available to each and every citizen the material, institutional, and educational circumstances in which good human functioning may be chosen; to move each and every one of them across a threshold of capability into circumstances in which they may choose to live and function well".

and nutrition, literacy, land rights, the right to seek employment outside the home, child marriage, and child labor" (Nussbaum, 2000, p. 7). In the dynamic raised by following or opposing John Rawls's (1972) political liberalism and the notion of "primary goods" combined with the economist Amartya Sen's approach on functioning and capability, she does not—in contrast to Sen (1987)—construe the Capabilities Approach as being provided with a comparative entity for standards of living but uses it "to articulate an account of how capabilities... can provide a basis for central constitutional principles that citizens have a right to demand from their governments" (Nussbaum, 2000, p. 12). What makes Nussbaum special is her formulation of a vague, open, arbitrarily extendable, politically relevant "list of functionings that is, on the one hand, non-detached, but, on the other hand, objective" (1988, p. 174). The functionings are considered to be equally fundamental without any hierarchy, although they exist at different levels.[4] Whereas, according to Nussbaum's judgement, bodily integrity is undeniably a basic capability, the inclusion of literacy in the list is doubtful in her eyes. Literacy is less timeless, it is "a concrete specification for the modern world of a more general capability that may have been realized without literacy in other times and places" (Nussbaum, 2000, pp. 77–78). Literacy is particularly formulated in the fourth[5] item of the list of central human capabilities as part of the following (Nussbaum, 2000):

Being able to use the senses, to imagine, think and reason—and to do these things in a "truly human" way, a way informed and cultivated by an adequate education, including, but by no means limited to, literacy and basic mathematical and scientific training. Being able to use imagination and thought in connection with experiencing, and producing self-expressive works and events of one's own choice, religious, literary, musical and so forth. Being able to use one's mind in ways protected by guarantees of freedom of expression with respect to both political and artistic speech, and freedom of religious exercise (pp. 78–79).

By postulating that capabilities must be supported and made possible, and that the individual's capabilities are indispensable for political and state tasks[6] while leaving the achieved functionings to the individual himself or herself, Nussbaum (1990, p. 224) formulates a universalistic approach that is able to take both pluralism and cultural differences into account to the same degree (Nussbaum, 1999, p. 202). This list does not claim to formulate a theory of justice. Instead, it is about defining a social minimum that a government must secure by way of social and political institutions (Nussbaum, 2000, p. 75).

---

[4]On the problem of the different capabilities levels, see also Pauer-Studer (1999, p. 21).

[5]The list of capabilities (Nussbaum, 2000, p. 78–80): (1) Life; (2) Bodily health; (3) Bodily integrity; (4) Senses, imagination and thought; (5) Emotions; (6) Practical reason; (7) Affiliation; (8) Other species; (9) Play; and (10) Control over one's environment: A. political, B. material

[6]"For now we are in a position to specify vaguely certain basic functionings that should, as constitutive of human life, concern us. We shall actually introduce the list as a list of the related capabilities, rather than of actual functionings, since we have argued that it is capabilities, not actual functionings, that should be in the legislator's goal" (Nussbaum, 1990, p. 224).

The relevance of Nussbaum's approach for the educational debate (see Albus, Andresen, Fegter, & Richter, 2009; Andresen, Otto, & Ziegler, 2008) on language education can be seen particularly on two levels: first, on the topical level of literacy, which is not defined closely by Nussbaum's concepts and is precisely not reduced to language capability.[7] Second, on the methodological level,[8] a particularly strong aspect of the Capabilities Approach is in being able to reconstruct and take into consideration both the individual-personal level and the political-institutional level when analysing the essential question of what someone "is actually able to do and to be" (Nussbaum, 2000, p. 71). "And we ask not just about the resources that are sitting around, but about how those do or do not go to work" (ibid.). Accordingly, the emphasis is on which resources are provided and how they are used to make human flourishing possible, or more concretely to secure that everybody has a choice to realize his/her own ideas of a "good life". In the following, on a theoretical level, we shall pursue the question of how language education could be described from the point of view of the Capabilities Approach and which incentives for language support might be derived from it.

3 Language Education as Making Capabilities Possible?

In our opinion, literacy, according to Nussbaum, works as an essential capability, in the sense of making all other capabilities possible or of initiating them. It serves as a precondition for most of the other items on Nussbaum's list. By literacy, we do not just refer to reading or writing skills or understanding and repeating the meaning of different texts. Instead, it represents a comprehensive language education that opens up access to the world via language while simultaneously making the individual's connection to the world possible. It addresses different sensory levels; it is relevant for imagination, thought and experiencing; and it includes the capability to deal communicatively with one's environment; just as, finally, it is considered to be the basic condition for political participation, self-determination and the possibility of influencing one's environment. This does not simply mean the subjective appropriation processes of children, but emphasizes the mutual relations.

In the German context, it does not seem to be self-evident that language education is more than learning the official language of German. For, even today being bi- and multi-lingual—despite more recent (education) policy proclamations—is associated with deficits and with growing up with deficits. Here, the debate on first and second

---

[7]Focusing on literacy in this article is not meant to give the impression that it is understood as a superior capability to other ones. This focus results exclusively from the research question. "In order to be doing what they should for their citizens, states must be concerned with all the capabilities" (Nussbaum, 2000, p. 90). This demand is not meant to be reduced here.

[8]Ingrid Robeyns (2005, p. 94) emphasises that "the capability approach is not a theory that can explain poverty, inequality or well-being, instead, it rather provides a tool and a framework within which to conceptualize and evaluate these phenomena".

language related to migration, which understands multilinguality as a resource, is able to change things only very slowly (see Leu, 2007; Mecheril & Quehl, 2006).

When referring to the concept of holism, all attempts at defining language education more closely make it quite different from linguistic positions that tend to be more interested in concepts of systematic language support. Holism, as Zehnbauer and Jampert (2007, p. 33) have expressed it, is that counter-position to linguistic concepts that goes back even to Pestalozzi and indicates that language support must be understood as an integrated part of the child's development of personality and appropriation of the environment. The concept of personality, they say, is one of the "(unquestioned) basic ideas of education" (ibid.). The joint framework decision of the Ministers for Youth from the year 2004 also refers to this explicitly: "The educational programme of Kindergartens is characterized by the principle of comprehensive support. The elementary level does not acknowledge any orientation towards subjects or scientific disciplines" (Beschluss der Jugendministerkonferenz Mai 2004, Beschluss der Kultusministerkonferenz Juni, 2004). This consensus includes accepting that language development in the sense of language education is understood as a unity of thinking, feeling and acting, as a multidimensional, stubborn, individual process, and in no way as a standardized, linear one (see Zehnbauer & Jampert, 2007, p. 34). From this point of view, the active and competent child according to more recent social-scientific childhood research (see Honig, 1999) is understood as an expert on his or her own development and as the constructor of his or her language acquisition, whose processes of language education are embedded at the Kindergarten into everyday situations of playing and acting and that, while following interactionist language theories, benefit particularly from adult-child dialogues (see Zehnbauer & Jampert, 2007).

The various country-specific educational plans formulated over the course of the past few years generally emphasize that language education at the elementary level is supposed to increase and support children's articulateness, making them able—in the sense of one competence resulting from the other—to develop their I-competencies, their social competencies, their factual competencies as well as those competencies related to literacy. In this context, one can find more or less concrete recommendations on how these educational goals could be implemented. However, the theoretical backgrounds, premises and implications remain mostly in the dark.[9]

Everything recently negotiated and defined under the keyword *language education* that refers to the premise of holism "means also the long-termedness and complexity of the development process and the didactic method, which does not serve any subject-specific small portions and turns against subject matter being exclusively communicated by adults" (Zehnbauer & Jampert, 2007, p. 35). Kindergarten educators are expected to be "highly sensitive towards the children's interests and needs", to "provide a language-friendly environment", to provide

---

[9]In this context, the curricula of the federal state of Hessen are a praiseworthy exception, in so far as they clearly document their social-constructivist and interaction-theoretical backgrounds (see Hessisches Sozialministerium/Hessisches Kultusministerium, 2005).

"consciously organized language support" by way of language inputs referring to everyday situations as well as by way of "purposeful work with small groups which, however, is embedded into the overall programme of the institution" (ibid.).

This way of understanding language education and the possibilities of supporting it seems to link up with the above understanding of literacy in the sense of a capability. According to the cornerstones summarized here, which give a holism-oriented definition of language education, "self-activity" proves to be an essential developmental, learning and also performance principle. Starting with this, it is about communicating processes that refer to "subjectively controlled perceptions" embedded into social contexts, to the child's "active dealing" with its environment. Following the Capabilities Approach, we argue that not only the subjective aspect is indispensable for the acquisition of language from the educational point of view, but that, most of all, the individual must be enabled to communicate by way of language, to make positions clear and to express them. This enabling must be encouraged performatively (Wulf & Zirfas, 2007) and in a dialogue context. In so far, outside situations play a key role. Also in the sense of Nussbaum, they serve as resources and necessary preconditions for the support of processes.

4 Conditions of Language Education—Reconstructed by Way of Participant Observation

As a direct response to the "PISA shock", German policy was to boost language support programmes and—preceding these—a variety of screening methods to measure the language skills of children at Kindergarten. There has been a boom in language interventions and, accordingly, of measurement methods to evaluate language skills. However, this has been accompanied by hardly any insights (see Albers, 2009): first, on how children at Kindergarten communicate with each other, how they make themselves understood and how they act; and second, on what kind of language support they experience in their daily lives (i.e. what communication towards them is like and which kinds of everyday-inclusive offers of language education are made to them). In the context of a research contract in the Rhine-Main area with the goal of delivering institution-specific analyses on language behaviour at kindergartens, a 1-week participant observation was conducted at each of three institutions with different catchment areas. One institution covered a socially mixed catchment area; the second, a socially disadvantaged neighbourhood; and the third had a rather middle- and upper-class clientele. Due to its design, this study made it possible to come close to the above-mentioned desideratum. It served the function of a pilot study. Its strong point was in putting the language-communicative milieu at individual kindergartens and the possibilities of language acquisition existing there into a characteristic light, and, starting out from this, in stimulating further ethnographic research. This study did not aim to comment on the language skills of individual children, as in a language skills diagnosis. Such a diagnosis, which refers exclusively to individual and selectively grasped language skills, is unable to assess the educational arrangement and the situational context of linguistic interaction. The educationally very reasonable question regarding whether or not an institution provides a milieu that is linguistically stimulating for children, cannot be answered with an individual-diagnostic method and an accordingly adjusted intervention practice aiming at controlled, systematic language acquisition but not at uncontrolled, group-related language acquisition. Instead, it is necessary to record the communicative contexts and situationally embedded linguistic interactions that are arranged educationally and conceptually at educational institutions. Our assumption was that observable everyday life, using materials, making group rules relevant and making ritualized processes necessary would reflect an institution's respective educational arrangement. In this sense, language and language acquisition may be considered essential factors of educational processes that are triggered by educational interventions in the context of the educational arrangement of the respective kindergarten, and that may be influenced from this perspective—in the context of which it will not be possible to answer the question whether and how children make use of such offers. Accordingly, our core research question was which language level is made possible by such varying contexts at Kindergarten. It has already been possible to give a basic answer to this question using one ethnographic method (Hirschauer & Amann, 1997): that of participant observation.[10] Therefore, ethnographic field notes (Emerson, Fretz, & Shaw, 1995) were taken and observation records were made.

Analyses of the records led to the identification of five different fields of language behaviour that are typical for everyday life at the Kindergarten: so-called conversation spaces. These are *periods in between*, unguided *free play*, *ritualized contexts*, *open offers*, as well as rather *segregating support situations*. These contexts differ clearly, on the one hand, in terms of the role behaviour of educators and children; on the other hand, in terms of language contents as well as ways of speaking. Moreover, they existed to different degrees or were weighted differently at all three institutions. After presenting the reconstructed characteristics of the first three conversation spaces, materials and contrasts will be used to discuss the contexts of *open offers* and *segregating support situations* in detail, because these contexts represent essential, structuring features of educational everyday life at two different institutions.

During the *period in between*, positioning and self-location within the space provide reasons to speak. The children do not just occupy certain places physically but also deal with their positions actively and verbally. Being a special kind of a period in between, arrival at Kindergarten may be described as a physicality- and adult-dominated transition dominated either by parents or by educators who provide reasons to speak.

Free game represents activities in situations that are not guided by educators. This context may be defined as the children's own realm; it is filled with their own

---

[10]The suitability of the method for kindergartens soon became obvious because the children quickly made contact with the observer and asked her what she was doing. They also used the presence of the observer as an opportunity to present self-made works of art to her and to stage themselves. They enjoyed observing the observer. Now and then—in a slightly controlling and also supporting mode—they asked her whether she had actually seen and noted this or that.

initiative and imagination. In this context, educators stay rather in the background, primarily they function as somebody providing help and as referees in conflict situations. Reasons to speak are unconventional actions requiring explanation, and most of all sensorily perceivable, presented materials. As a result, the materials with which the Kindergarten is equipped are particularly relevant for language education. On the basis of sensorily perceivable objects, children start associations and thus initiate a topic to be discussed by the group. Children's associative way of speaking becomes particularly obvious in free-game situations. During free game periods, the children linguistically accompany and comment on their current and previous actions. The topical emphasis of the children's statements is on ownership ("that's mine"), performance ("I can do this on my own"), needs ("I need another red coloured pencil!"), social and language behaviour, what they are or are not allowed to do and say as well as talking about what they are doing at the moment.

Ritualized contexts (such as sitting in a circle to start the Kindergarten day, sitting in the good-bye circle, weekly walks or the rituals connected with eating together) structure everyday life at all three kindergartens to different degrees. These contexts are primarily characterized by their function of creating a community. The difference to other everyday actions is construed by the framework of the rituals: the arrangement of the environments belonging to the respective ritual like place, time and collectivity (Turner, 1989; Wulf, 2008). Ritualized contexts at kindergarten are most of all staged by forming a circle. An analysis of the records made at all three institutions clearly shows a paradox of this circle situation: the paradox of subjectivation and desubjectivation processes, of staging and presenting, that is, the fact that although each child is given the opportunity to stage himself or herself, this situation includes a presentation demand that may particularly overtax the youngest children.

We called *open offers* all those educator-initiated and consciously stimulated voluntary contexts offered to all children and also across groups. Looking at the social structure, the catchment area of one kindergarten was mostly upper middle class. According to the deputy head's appraisal, this institution was provided with sufficient staff and had sufficient resources to provide many creative support provisions for the children or together with the children that are integrated into everyday life. Being oriented towards a semi-open concept, the institution used a great deal of cross-group activities and projects that were also jointly planned in the context of the so-called children's parliament. Apart from classrooms, the day nursery had rooms for special activities with different emphases, with a physical training hall, a crafts room, a room for English lessons as well as a library offering nonfiction books, fairytale books and picture books, where work was also carried out in small groups with children of preschool age. To illustrate our research method and to give an idea of everyday life at Kindergarten, the following passage from a record is analysed below:

"Who would like to listen to The Very Hungry Caterpillar[11]" an educator asks the children in the "Rabbit" Class. "Me, me", the children shout. "And what about you, Mareike, would

[11] The very popular German translation of Eric Carle's (1969) world-famous book is Kleine Raupe Nimmersatt.

you like to listen to the story?" the educator asks one girl. "I've got a book on it", the girl replies. "That's beautiful. You might help me with telling the story", the educator says. The girl nods. "I know this story", one boy shouts. "Me too" another child says. "In the cellar, I have already prepared something for telling the story. If you like, you can go downstairs, I shall just ask the other children", the educator explains. Downstairs, she starts talking at a very low voice. "Do you see the moon?" she asks the children, who are sitting in a circle around a big blanket. The children point at a white, round cloth which is placed above, at the "sky".

Here, the educator presents an open offer to the children. The criterion for taking part in this literary-inspired story offer is "to like". A general, harmless category that attributes the feature "interested" and not the feature "in need of support" to the children. Nevertheless, not only those children who like are addressed by this suggestion, for the educator individually addresses other children and tries to convince them. By presenting arguments, she starts a conversation with the children and tries to win them over for her offer. Questions are made transparent in a latent and recognisable way. After the group of listeners has been put together, the children in this "story room" are integrated into the story by the educator's attention-guiding questions. Because they are sitting on the ground, the children have more freedom to move and more possibilities to intervene, also physically, bodily, in the story. During the course of the story, the children, while "acting" the story, equip the blue blanket with toy figures, pieces of cloth and plastic fruits. The youngest are given the opportunity to make butterflies out of glass and decorative stones to illustrate the story. The story was co-constructed and re-acted interactively using a range of different materials to stimulate sensory perception.

Segregating support situations is what we call different, binding offers intended for and offered to one defined group selected according to certain features (such as age, migration background, sex). The educators initiate, guide and coordinate the interactions that, for the example of language support, include exercises on phonologic awareness, but no conversations. In these situations, different tactics are applied so that the children work out a free space for themselves that forms the basis for further discussions and conversations among each other.

One of the three institutions placed a strong emphasis on supporting movement and language, particularly for children with a migration background. This support was arranged by segregating certain subgroups and took an everyday-structuring nature. It was mostly socially disadvantaged families who lived in the catchment area of this kindergarten. Whereas the proportion of children with a migration background was rather low at the two other kindergartens, it was more than 50% here. The institution also promoted a semi-open concept. There was a wide hall containing a miniature kitchen, a piano and the table soccer with the classrooms, the recreation room, bathrooms, sports room and crafts room leading off it. This space served as an exchange centre for the children. A painting studio had been set up between two rooms. It was notable that books were placed on the upper shelves in the hall and in some of the classrooms as well, so that the children needed help from an adult to reach them. An excerpt from the following one scene at lunchtime illustrates the value of language support:

> The educator places herself directly behind Francesco, with the boy's hands, she holds the cutlery, knocks on the table with the knife and fork and says: "This fork! This knife! You must not always cry. You must learn that. If he always drinks from the bottle, he will not learn it", she finally tells the other children. "If you want more, you get up and get some", the educator says towards Francesco.

This scene makes the educator's normative behaviour particularly obvious through the use of passive constructions and the auxiliary verb "must". Such directing sentence constructions do not allow room for any doubts, questions, comments or other ways of behaving. Both the way in which the educator speaks and the way in which she behaves towards—most of all—Francesco are of a domineering, even violent nature. The educator legitimizes this way of speaking by the necessity of "being obliged to speak German". In this scene, in an educational context in which more than 50% of the children had a migration background, the German language is made the absolute basic category of mutual understanding and being able to communicate. By not allowing for or not accepting any other further means of communication—such as other languages or bodily gestures—everything that is not stated in German is devalued and discriminated. Even the boy's crying seems to be incomprehensible. What makes the situation paradoxical is the use of grammatically incomplete[12] sentences as well as a hierarchical, nonappreciative and not at all supportive atmosphere due to the authoritarian way of speaking dominated by orders.

If the starting point is the question in the Capabilities Approach regarding what someone "is actually able to do and to be" (Nussbaum, 2000, p. 71), we recognise that children from disadvantaged social classes and minority groups need more material support from public institutions than those from the middle and upper classes if they are to have equal access to education (Nussbaum, 1990, p. 211). Thus, it is even more astonishing that it is precisely the Kindergarten frequented by more children from socially disadvantaged classes that has the least staff and material resources. We may assume that such conditions are less favourable for language education, and from the point of view of creating, supporting and securing equal opportunities of education at and by educational institutions, they will not contribute much. Indeed, we can assume the exact opposite: They not only confirm but also reproduce the existing social (dis)order.

5 Conclusion and Prospects

In the German context, the Capabilities Approach in Nussbaum's sense is sometimes called the "enabling approach" (*Befähigungsansatz*, Oelkers & Schrödter, 2008; Otto & Ziegler, 2008). This means that it is a theoretical-normative frame for not only the individual's development processes but also conditions or resources, in

---

[12]The sentences were incomplete in the German version, because the educator dropped the definite articles when naming the objects knife and fork ("Das ist Messer! Das ist Gabel!").

other words, the opportunity spaces provided by the environment. In our opinion, what makes the Capabilities Approach special is the combination of individual-personal and political-institutional aspects in the sense of creating and enabling conditions for success. From educational and pedagogical points of view, it seems to be more than relevant to examine both the individual and, on the outside, the external structural conditions when addressing issues in how to bring up and educate children. The concept of literacy as a capability in Nussbaum's sense, which we apply synonymously to the concept of language education presented here, requires a minimum of outside, arranged material and staff conditions to have its full effect. The individual must be able to fall back on these conditions in order to unleash his or her potential.

The research approach presented here was based on a concept of language education that is supposed to include more than language support. Accordingly, the focus was not on the subjective acquisition processes of individual children but on enabling contexts at kindergarten. The micro-analysis of communicative practices opens up the access to educationally arranged everyday events and makes them empirically accessible, reconstructable and evaluable in terms of the resources they provide for children in relation to processes of language acquisition, which, in the sense of the Capabilities Approach, are considered to be the basic condition for later political participation, self-determination and possibilities to not only influence but also deal communicatively with one's environment.

References

Albers, T. (2009). *Sprache und Interaktion im Kindergarten. Eine quantitativ-qualitative Analyse der sprachlichen und kommunikativen Kompetenzen von drei- bis sechsjährigen Kindern.* Klinkhardt, Bad Heilbrunn, Germany.

Albus, S., Andresen, S., Fegter, S., & Richter, M. (2009): Wohlergehen und das "gute Leben" in der Perspektive von Kindern. Das Potenzial des Capability Approach für die Kindheitsfroschung. *Zeitschrift für Soziologie der Erziehung und Sozialisation, 29*(4), 346–358.

Andresen, S., Otto, H.-U., & Ziegler, H. (2008). Bildung as human development: An educational view on the capabilities approach. In H.-U. Otto & H. Ziegler (Eds.), *Capabilities – Handlungsbefähigung und Verwirklichungschancen in der Erziehungswissenschaft* (pp. 165–198). Wiesbaden: VS-Verlag.

Apeltauer, E. (2007). Sprachliche Frühförderung von Kindern mit Migrationshintergrund. *Info DaF, 34*(1), 3–36.

Beschluss der Kultusministerkonferenz Juni. (2004). Beschluss der Jugendminister vom 13./14. Mai 2004 und Beschluss der Kultusminister vom 3./4. Juni 2004: Gemeinsamer Rahmen der Länder für die frühe Bildung in Kindertageseinrichtungen. Accessed December 2009, from www.kmk.org/filadmin/veroeffentlichungen_beschluesse/2004/2004_06_04-Fruehe-Bildung-Kitas.pdf

Carle, E. (1969). Die kleine Raupe Nimmersatt, Gerstenberg Verlag, Hildesheim, Germany.

Emerson, R. M., Fretz, R. I., & Shaw, L. L. (1995). *Writing ethnographic fieldnotes.* Chicago: Chicago University Press.

Hessisches Sozialministerium/Hessisches Kultusministerium (Ed.). (2005). *Bildung von Anfang an. Bildungs- und Erziehungsplan für Kinder von 0 bis 10 Jahren in Hessen.* Broschüre Stand März 2005, Wiesbaden.

Hirschauer, S., & Amann, K. (1997). Die Befremdung der eigenen Kultur. Ein Programm. In S. Hirschauer & K. Amann (Eds.), *Die Befremdung der eigenen Kultur. Zur ethnographischen Herausforderung soziologischer Empirie* (pp. 7–52). Frankfurt am Main: Suhrkamp.

Honig, M.-S. (1999): *Entwurf einer Theorie der Kindheit*. Frankfurt am Main: Suhrkamp.

Leu, H. R. (2007). Die Bildungsdebatte in Deutschland – heute und vor dreißig Jahren, Gemeinsamkeiten und Unterschiede. In K. Jampert, P. Best, A. Guadatiello, D. Holler, & A. Zehnbauer (Eds.), *Schlüsselkompetenz Sprache. Sprachliche Bildung und Förderung im Kindergarten, Konzepte, Projekte und Maßnahmen* (pp. 19–23). Weimar, Berlin: Verlag das netz.

Lütje-Klose, B. (2007). Sprachstandserhebungen im Vorschulalter. In T. Fleischer, N. Grewe, B. Jötten, & K. Seifried (Eds.), *Handbuch der Schulpsychologie, Psychologie für die Schule* (pp. 133–144). Stuttgart: Kohlhammer.

Mecheril, P., & Quehl, T. (Eds.). (2006). *Die Macht der Sprachen: Englische Perspektiven auf die mehrsprachige Schule*. Münster: Waxmann.

Nussbaum, M. C. (1988). Nature, function, and capability: Aristotle on political distribution. *Oxford Studies in Ancient Philosophy*, Supplemental Volume, 145–184.

Nussbaum, M. C. (1990). Aristotelian social democracy. In R. B. Douglas, G. Mara, & H. Richardson (Eds.), *Liberalism and the good* (pp. 203–252). New York: Routledge.

Nussbaum, M. C. (1999). In H. Pauer-Studer (Ed.), *Gerechtigkeit oder Das gute Leben* (pp. 176–226). Frankfurt am Main: Suhrkamp.

Nussbaum, M. C. (2000). *Women and human development. The capabilities approach*. Cambridge: Cambridge University Press.

Nussbaum, M. C. (2005). Well-being, contracts and capabilities. In L. Manderson (Ed.), *Rethinking well-being* (pp. 27–44). Perth: API Network.

Oelkers, N., & Schrödter, M. (2008). Soziale Arbeit im Dienste der Befähigungsgerechtigkeit. In Bielefelder Arbeitsgruppe 8 (Ed.), *Soziale Arbeit in Gesellschaft* (pp. 44–49). Wiesbaden: VS-Verlag.

Otto, H.-U., & Ziegler, H. (2008). Der Capabilities-Ansatz als neue Orientierung in der Erziehungswissenschaft. In H.-U. Otto & H. Ziegler (Eds.), *Capabilities – Handlungsbefähigung und Verwirklichungschancen in der Erziehungswissenschaft* (pp. 9–16). Wiesbaden: VS-Verlag.

Pauer-Studer, H. (1999). Einleitung. In M. C. Nussbaum (Ed.), *Gerechtigkeit oder Das gute Leben* (pp. 7–23). Frankfurt am Main: Suhrkamp.

Rawls, J. (1972). *A theory of justice*. Oxford: Clarendon Press.

Robeyns, I. (2005). The capability approach: A theoretical survey. *Journal of Human Development and Capabilities*, 6(1), 93–117.

Sen, A. (1987). *The standard of living*. Cambridge: Cambridge University Press.

Turner, V. (1989). *Das Ritual. Struktur und Anti-Struktur*. Frankfurt am Main: Campus.

Wulf, C. (2008). Rituale im Grundschulalter: Performativität, Mimesis und Interkulturalität. *Zeitschrift für Erziehungswissenschaft*, 11(1), 67–83.

Wulf, C., & Zirfas, J. (2007). Performative Pädagogik und performative Bildungstheorien. Ein neuer Fokus erziehungswissenschaftlicher Forschung. In C. Wulf & J. Zirfas (Eds.), *Pädagogik des Performativen. Theorien, Methoden, Perspektiven* (pp. 7–12). Weinheim: Beltz.

Zehnbauer, A., & Jampert, K. (2007). Sprachliche Bildung und Sprachförderung im Rahmen einer ganzheitlichen Elementarpädagogik. In K. Jampert, P. Best, A. Guadatiello, D. Holler, & A. Zehnbauer (Eds.), *Schlüsselkompetenz Sprache. Sprachliche Bildung und Förderung im Kindergarten, Konzepte, Projekte und Maßnahmen* (pp. 33–37). Weimar, Berlin: Verlag das netz.

Part III
Children's Perspectives: Methodological Critiques and Empirical Studies

Christine Hunner-Kreisel and Melanie Kuhn

1 Introduction

Listening to what children say about their lives, their dreams and their sorrows—respectively their well-being—has become almost a methodological paradigm in western approaches to the study of children and their life worlds (Ben-Arieh, 2005; Ben-Arieh et al., 2001; Honig, 1999a). The current tradition in childhood studies focusing on children as competent actors and experts on their own lives is also reflected in recent studies in which children are addressed either as main informants (Mayall, 1994; Wilk, 1996; World Vision, 2007) or they are "given a voice" by including their standpoints as part of the data collection (UNICEF, 2007, p. 5). Nevertheless, there are still studies that do not incorporate children as resources of information (NICHD, 2005).

As part of the methodological shift in childhood studies, even very young children have been incorporated in research. The so-called "Mosaic-Approach" by Alison Clark and Peter Moss is an innovative and creative methodological approach to research with very small children (Clark & Moss, 2001, p. 6) in which children use a camera, lead tours and design maps of the places in their worlds, thereby offering—combined with so-called child conferences, interviews or observation—a deeper understanding of their perspectives on their own lifeworlds. The data collected is further complemented from the parents' perspectives by asking them the same questions the children have been asked and interviewing them on the subjects their children have thought important (Clark & Moss, 2001, p. 32).

The new research paradigm with its main interest in the children's view developed in opposition to the sciences of socialisation and developmental psychology. The latter focused upon children mainly as persons who still have to grow up and are therefore "adults to be". Criticising this view on children the scientific way of exploring the "perspective of the child" was given free. But, what is the

C. Hunner-Kreisel (✉)
Faculty of Educational Science, Bielefeld University, 33615 Bielefeld, Germany
e-mail: christine.hunner-kreisel@uni-bielefeld.de

methodological and epistemological meaning of the phrase "from the perspective of the child"? As Honig, Lange and Leu (1999) have argued, this guiding theme in the current tradition of childhood studies seems to be more of a programmatic agreement than a reasoned methodological construct. By overemphasising the subjective perspective of children, childhood research is possibly in danger of failing to register the appearance of adaptive preferences (Clark, 2009; Elster, 1983; Lugo & Samman, 2008; Sen, 1985a, b) and thereby overlooking the structural conditions of growing up. For the field of childhood studies, the methodological problem of adaptive preferences is predicated on the phenomenon that the spectrum of childhood desires, life expectations and their satisfaction may well adapt to the available structural, economical and political options. Especially the field of so-called "happiness" research, with its main focus on the aspect of subjective well-being, is therefore at risk of taking subjective feelings of joy as its basic indicator. Childhood research has to go beyond investigating the subjective ideas and feelings of the child actor. Otherwise, it will run the risk of neglecting social inequality and injustice (see also Marks, Sha & Westall, 2004; Nussbaum, 2000; Otto & Ziegler, 2007; Sen, 1985a, b, 1990). Children also have to be seen within the institutional and societal boundaries defining the space within which they can act. Following these premises, the study of childhood(s) has to be accompanied by analyses of class, race and gender as well as the framework of historical, social and cultural backgrounds (Alanen, 1992; Alanen & Bardy, 1991; Butterwegge, Klundt & Belke-Zeng, 2008; Honig, 1999b; James, Jenks & Prout, 1998; Lareau, 2003; Qvortrup, 1992; Vincent & Ball, 2006).

Focusing only on the "perspective of the child" raises even more problems. One main point is the question of the constitutive representation of the "child's voice" by an adult researcher. The hidden implications of the slogan "giving children a voice" are to make children socially visible and provide an auditorium for them on a political level (Lipski, 2000, p. 420). At the same time, this reveals the normative and sometimes paternalistic moral standpoint of broad sections of this kind of childhood research. To achieve the aim of doing research not about but *from the perspective* of children, the current tradition of childhood studies mostly postulates the need for an intense and democratic integration of children in all stages of the research process. Nonetheless, such participation strategies have to be scrutinised to see whether they are more than just a naive effort to use children's participation to capture an expression of children's voices that is as *authentic* as possible. This would be based in a foreshortened manner on the assumption that identity produces knowledge in a determined way. And in this sense, children would automatically have a privileged access to childhood experience and knowledge—based on their identity. According to this, participation would naturally cause a privileged representation. By following this way of thinking, as Bühler-Niederberger (2007) has been pointing out, children have become essentialised naively and constructed in an outline view as being mostly different from adults. As a result, participatory strategies will hardly make structurally given power imbalances between adult researchers and children as subjects of the research (Christensen, 2004) disappear. A better approach is to reflect on and analyse them as part of the generational order (Alanen, 1992). In this sense, "the children's perspective is no reality, which could be discovered or described through research. The children's perspective is rather a structural characteristic of the relation between child and adult" (Honig, 1999a, p. 45, translated).

Any simple participation of children as authentic informants seems to be even more complex against the background of power imbalances, because, due to social background, not every child possesses the same resources (Melton & Limber, 1992) and, as a result, the same capabilities or agency (James, 2009) to represent himself or herself and his or her worlds in the process of research. These critical considerations can be found in some older debates in ethnology and anthropology on the topic of substitutional representation. The aim of grasping and representing the so-called "native point of view" is criticised clearly and broadly for its powerful constructions of an essentially different "other" and for its insufficient regard to power imbalances between researcher and the subjects of research (Berg & Fuchs, 1993; Clifford & Marcus, 1986). This fundamental critique of the representation of "the other" should make us aware that childhood research—even when it aims to be research from the perspective of the children—inevitably produces images and knowledge over children und childhood as well.

References

Alanen, L. (1992). *Modern childhood? Exploring the "child question*. Sociology Research Reports Vol. 50. University of Jyväskylä, Finland, Institute of Educational Research.

Alanen, L., & Bardy, M. (1991). *Childhood as a social phenomenon*. Vienna: European Centre for Social Welfare Policy and Research.

Ben-Arieh, A. (2005). Where are the children? Children's role in measuring and monitoring their well-being. *Social Indicators Research, 74*(3), 573–596.

Ben-Arieh, A., Hevener Kaufmann, N., Bowers, A., Goerge, R. M., Lee, B. J., & Aber, J. L. (2001). *Measuring and monitoring children's well-being*. Dordrecht: Kluwer.

Berg, E., & Fuchs, M. (Eds.). (1993). *Kultur, soziale Praxis, Text: Die Krise der ethnographischen Repräsentation*. Frankfurt a. M.: Suhrkamp.

Bühler-Niederberger, D. (2007). *The power of innocence. Social politics for children between separation and participation*. Institute of Childhood and Urban World. (Wellchi Working Paper Series, No. 4). doi: www.ciimu.org/webs/wellchi/publications.htm

Butterwegge, C., Klundt, M., & Belke-Zeng, M. (2008). *Kinderarmut in Ost- und Westdeutschland*. Wiesbaden: VS-Verlag für Sozialwissenschaften.

Christensen, P. (2004). Children's participation in ethnographic research: Issues of power and representation. *Children and Society, 18*, 165–176.

Clark, D. (2009). *Adaption, poverty and wellbeing: Some issues and observations with special reference to the capability approach and development studies*. (Working Paper 081). University of Manchester, England: Global Poverty Research Group. Accessed November 25, 2009, from http://www.gprg.org/pubs/work ingpapers/pdfs.gprg-wps-081.pdf

Clark, A., & Moss, P. (2001). *Listening to young children. The mosaic approach*. London: National Children's Bureau.

Clifford, J., & Marcus, G. E. (1986). *Writing culture. The poetics and politics of ethnography*. Berkeley, CA: University of California Press.

Elster, J. (1983). *Sour grapes: Studies in the subversion of rationality*. Cambridge: Cambridge University Press.

Honig, M.-S. (1999a). Forschung "vom Kinde aus"? Perspektivität in der Kindheitsforschung. In M.-S. Honig, A. Lange, & H. R. Leu (Eds.), *Aus der Perspektive von Kindern? Zur Methodologie der Kindheitsforschung* (pp. 33–50). Weinheim: Juventa.

Honig, M.-S., Lange, A., & Leu, H. R. (1999). Eigenart und Fremdheit. Kindheitsforschung und das Problem der Differenz von Kindern und Erwachsenen. In M.-S. Honig, A. Lange, & H. R. Leu (Eds.), *Aus der Perspektive von Kindern? Zur Methodologie der Kindheitsforschung* (pp. 9–32). Weinheim: Juventa.

James, A. (2009). Agency. In J. Qvortrup, W. A. Corsaro, & M.-S. Honig (Eds.), *The Palgrave handbook of childhood studies* (pp. 34–46). Basingstoke: Palgrave Macmillan.

James, A., Jenks, C., & Prout, A. (1998). *Theorizing childhood*. Cambridge: Polity Press.

Lareau, A. (2003). *Unequal childhoods: Class, race and family life*. Berkeley, CA: University of California Press.

Lipski, J. (2000). Kindern eine Stimme geben. Erfahrungen mit sozialwissenschaftlichen Kinderbefragungen. Giving children a voice. *Zeitschrift für Soziologie der Erziehung und Sozialisation, 18*(4), 403–422.

Lugo, M. A., & Samman, E. (2008). *An empirical exploration of integrating subjective health perceptions into multidimensional capability measures*. Paper prepared for the 30th General Conference of The International Association for Research in Income and Wealth, Portoroz, Slovenia.

Marks, N., Sha, H., & Westall, A. (2004). *The power and potential of well-being indicators. Measuring young people's well-being in Nottingham*. London: NEF.

Mayall, B. (Ed.). (1994). *Children's childhoods: Observed and experienced*. London: Routledge Falmer.

Melton, G. B., & Limber, S. P. (1992). What rights mean to children: Cross-cultural perspectives. In P. Veerman (Ed.), *Ideologies of children's rights*. Dordrecht: Martinus Nijhoff.

NICHD Early Child Care Research Network (Ed.). (2005). *Child care and child development: Results from the NICHD study of early child care and youth development*. New York: Guilford Press.

Nussbaum, M. (2000). *Women and human development*. Cambridge: Cambridge University Press.

Otto, H.-U., & Ziegler, H. (2007). Soziale Arbeit, Glück und das gute Leben. In S. Andresen, I. Pinhard, & S. Weyers (Eds.), *Erziehung – Ethik – Erinnerung* (pp. 229–248). Weinheim: Beltz.

Qvortrup, J. (1992). *Childhood as a social phenomenon: An introduction to a series of national reports*. Vienna: European Centre for Social Welfare Policy and Research.

Sen, A. K. (1985a). *Commodities and capabilities*. Amsterdam: North Holland.

Sen, A. K. (1985b). *The standard of living: The Tanner lectures*. Cambridge: Cambridge University Press.

Sen, A. K. (1990). Justice. Means versus freedoms. *Philosophy and Public Affairs, 19*, 111–12

UNICEF (2007). *The state of the world's children 2007*. New York: UNICEF House.

Vincent, C., & Ball, S. J. (2006). *Childcare, choice and class practices. Middle-class parents and their children*. London: Routledge.

Wilk, L. (1996). Die Studie "Kindsein in Österreich". Kinder und ihre Lebenswelten als Gegenstand empirischer Sozialforschung – Chancen und Grenzen einer Surveyerhebung. In M.-S. Honig, H. R. Leu, & U. Nissen (Eds.), *Kinder und Kindheit. Soziokulturelle Muster – sozialisationstheoretische Perspektiven* (pp. 55–76). Weinheim: Juventa.

World Vision Deutschland (Ed.). (2007). *Kinder in Deutschland 2007. 1. World Vision Kinderstudie*. Frankfurt am Main: Fischer.

Biographical Research in Childhood Studies: Exploring Children's Voices from a Pedagogical Perspective

Gonzalo Jover and Bianca Thoilliez

1 Introduction

In this chapter, we present a line of research being carried out over the last 12 years by the Research Group on Pedagogy of Children's Values from the *Universidad Complutense de Madrid* (Spain).[1] In 1997, with the financial support of the *Fundación Crecer Jugando* ("Growing Through Playing Foundation"), we started a line focused on listening to children's voices. Our interest is in education, so by studying what children believe, say and imagine, we intended not only to find out what those voices reveal but also to make recommendations for educational practice.

Our first attempt, entitled *The World of the Child* (*I*) (Gil & Jover, 2000), was a pilot project delving into the possibilities of narrative approaches in child education. The specific objective of the research was to use a biographical methodology to analyse how primary school children (aged 6–12 years) perceive the world they live in and the world they would like to have. After that, *The Right to Education*: *Worldwide Prospects* was carried out in 1998 (Jover, 2001). This research explored the legal, ethical and pedagogical aspects of the right to education. It aimed to find out the global attitudes towards this right. To that end, advances in information and communication technologies were used to distribute a brief questionnaire with four open-ended questions. The questionnaire was then sent over the Internet in four languages: Spanish, English, French and German. Information about the study was e-mailed to more than 600 international organizations, universities and associations involved in human rights, education, childhood development, women's rights and cultural awareness from all over the world.

That same year, we carried out the educational experience *Growing with Rights* in 16 Spanish primary schools (Gil & Jover, 1998) with more than 700 pupils aged 10–12 years and 30 teachers. The project was based on the idea that children's rights

G. Jover (✉)
Faculty of Education, Complutense University of Madrid, Ciudad Universitaria,
28040 Madrid, Spain
e-mail: gjover@edu.ucm.es

[1] http://www.ucm.es/info/quiron/pedinfant/

S. Andresen et al. (eds.), *Children and the Good Life*, Children's Well-Being: Indicators and Research 4, DOI 10.1007/978-90-481-9219-9_9,
© Springer Science+Business Media B.V. 2010

aim to promote the image of boys and girls as active agents. Thus, when teaching rights, we must start by having an open dialogue on the personal experience children have about their own rights. Our next project was *Images of the Other in Childhood* (1999), which attempted to understand how children represent others (Jover & Reyero, 2000). Based on a methodological design suggested by cultural studies and visual anthropology, the project sought to answer the question "What do children see in the images of those who are culturally different?" From this project, we concluded that educating in a multicultural environment means teaching to see the relativity and artificiality of cultural borders, helping to find the "you" living in the other—the biography of a particular individual beyond tags and labels.

In 2001, we then carried out *Peace Education: Life Behind Images* (Gil, Jover, & Reyero, 2003). The main aim was to determine how Spanish children imagine other children in war, how they think their lives are. Some ideas on educating for peace in the light of child narrative constructions were then suggested. The proposals of moral education for peace usually try to promote feelings and attitudes of solidarity and empathy towards others. The results of our research showed that promoting knowledge is also needed for children to become aware of reality in order to understand the reasons for human conflicts. Following that, *Children's Perception of Constitutional Values* was a piece of research we carried out in 2003 (Gil & Jover, 2003) to discover how teenagers live and experience the higher values that sustain civic life in a democratic society. Once again, we used methodologies based on images and narratives. The project provided suggestions for improving ways of understanding and designing civic education programmes. The aim of *Remembering Toys* (2005) was to analyse from a pedagogical point of view the memories of four generations about TV commercials for toys and games (Gil, Jover, & Reyero, 2006). Advertisements for toys and games from the 1960s onwards were used. The participants belonged to four different generations: those who were children in 1960, 1975, 1990 and 2005. One of the main conclusions was that toys and games play an important role in the current tendency to retreat into increasingly narrow spaces of socialization.

Our last two projects are *The World of the Child (II)* and *Growing Happy*. The first one is presented here. The second one is currently underway; we have recently finished the field work, so we shall focus on the methodological design.

2 Biographical Research with Children: The World of the Child (II)

The rise of biographical research is set within what some authors call the "narrative turn" that has been taken in the knowledge of education. This turn has led to a rediscovery of the subjects' own life experiences, in sharp contrast to the objectivist attempts of positivist methodologies in which the educator and the student are treated as replaceable representatives of some prototype. Thus, rather than being a specific research method, in pedagogic circles, the narrative and biographical approach is considered a paradigm, a new way of understanding education and pedagogical knowledge, that fans out into different lines of research.

One of the fields in which this approach has been applied the most since the late 1970s—for both research and training—is initial and ongoing teacher education. Its application to learners, however, has focused chiefly on the adult population, adult education and students of higher education. Far less exploration has been made of its possibilities in the area of early childhood education. Our research tried to fill this gap.

3 Methodological Design

One fairly common characteristic among the different lines of work involving the narrative approach in education is the frequent fusion of biography as a research method and biography as a method of teaching and education. We adopted this double orientation. The purpose of the research was to capture the life experience of primary school children (aged 6–12) from the point of view of their perception as subjects. The basic question we were trying to answer is how these children experience the world they live in, where "world" means both their proximal realm of experience (school, family, friends etc.) and the realm of global experience (the world in the broader sense and their place in it). At the same time, we hoped to check the pedagogical value of biographical methodology by means of an example of its use in the classroom.

We employed a technique of multiple and thematic life stories. The subjects lending their voice to the research were 40 children (consisting of 20 boys and 20 girls) with ages ranging from 6 to 12 years, from five public and private schools distributed across different parts of Spain. Data were collected with written stories and in-depth, open, biographical interviews. The protocol for the interview included five categories or broad topics of analysis: my family, my school, my friends, me myself and the world I imagine.

The information-gathering process began through prior contact with each collaborating school in which one person was assigned as to take charge of the initial phases. This person was given a guideline paper with the details of the research, an individualized record card for each child (to gather information on the child's family situation and any other circumstantial information) and a summary card on the school.

The procedure to follow in the initial phase depended on whether the participant belonged to the lower (6–9 years) or higher (10–12 years) age group. The younger group was asked to take their time and draw a picture of each of two topics: (a) my family, and (b) the world as I imagine it is. The drawings were collected and sent to the research team along with each child's record card. The older children were asked to write a short story on the same two topics of analysis above. The rest of the process remained the same.

The research team then used this material to prepare an individualized interview with each child. All interviews were recorded. The recordings and the stories written by the older children constituted the material for analysing the information. We based this on the *grounded theory* approach, which is considered best suited to the multiple story technique we used.

3.1 Results

As Bruner says, "no text can be interpreted on only one level" (Bruner, 1996, p. 17). The same is true of biographical stories. A sociologist, an anthropologist, a psychologist and a pedagogue will not find the same things in the children's stories. What interest can they have from a pedagogical point of view? Our proposal is to see these stories as manifestations of the *ethical experience of being in the world*. As is customary in qualitative research, this key of interpretation is a general criterion to guide the interpretation, and not a closed working hypothesis.

We shall adhere to the following sequence of topics when discussing the results: self, family, school, friends and the world. All the names used to identify the children have been changed, keeping only the original age and gender of each author.

(A) Self

The description given by the children when speaking of themselves is a combination of physical, biographical and moral traits. These descriptions reveal the tension between being and should be. This tension comes to the forefront more in the realm of the home than the school. Juan, 6 years old, is quite explicit. He says that at home he is a little more unruly than at school, because

> When I'm at home, I set traps to make sure nobody gets into my room. . . I tie a rope to the bed, to the foot, and another rope to the radiator, to that part underneath it, to the foot of the radiator, when someone tries to come in, bam! it slams in their face. I yell "Don't come in" and they come in. . . My mom says I'm bad. . . At school, I don't have stuff to set traps, no ropes, no nothing.

The children readily acknowledge that their behaviour is sometimes inappropriate, and they show none of the adult's need for self-justification.

Life at these ages starts expanding quickly from the past into the present and future. The past becomes part of personal experience. In their stories, the children often refer to key moments in their past, normally exceptional moments: an important change in their way of life or some moment when, for some reason, they became the centre of family attention. The present chiefly involves life and everyday worries: problems with friends, relationships at home or the situation at school. From our adult perspective, the problems they tell about can seem insignificant. Taking children seriously means understanding that for them, these problems are significant parts of their current experience. Last, the future is aspirations, hopes and what seems to take too long to come. The tension towards the future takes its models from the known adult world. When asked what they want to be when they grow up, they refer to well-known things, things normally found in their surroundings. And, at times, they are not very clear on just what that world consists of. Thus, some children say they want to enter some professions even though they are unsure of what those professions entail. But that is their least concern. For them, the most important thing is to approach the model, the lifestyle their choice embodies.

(B) Family

The family represents the realm of safety and affective ties. The children's stories depict the various typologies of families. The family is a place for life in common and for learning about collaboration. The allocation of roles follows the traditional schema. Normally, it is the mothers who take the children to school when they are small, who help them with their homework and who take care of them when they are sick. The father still represents the authority figure. For most children, relations with brothers and sisters are the first experience of disputes over conflicts of interest. For the children, continual fighting does not mean disaffection; rather, it is lived as everyday experiences of tension for self-assertion.

Home also represents the first experience with solitude, with experiencing absence. The parents are often experienced as absent figures. The experience of absence may be a consequence of certain current social conditions, but, in a deeper sense, it is also a sign of the cultural orientation towards independence. In this orientation, emancipation and breaking ties are valued as signs of growth.

(C) School

In their stories and comments, the children take attending school as a positive experience that sometimes seems to represent an escape route from the monotony of family life, especially, it seems, as children get older. School, and the school playground in particular, are experienced as an environment for relationships, for discovering the other and for conflict. For some children, school also represents the opportunity for the moral experience of taking care of the other. Ana, 12 years old, explained it to us in the following way:

> Because, since there are all kinds of people who you meet, and that's why, for example there's a girl who's in a wheelchair and she doesn't talk a lot, but for me, if do things to make them happy, they make me happy.

In teachers, the children most prize their affective qualities and politeness. They want them to be nice, and above all, not to yell at them. Along with these traits, children also value some pedagogic qualities, such as teaching ability, helpfulness and pedagogical tact.

The negative aspects of school life are usually associated with difficulties in learning some subject matter, homework and sanctions. They also include a few rather unpedagogic attitudes the children pick up from how they are treated by their teachers. Carmen, 8 years old, told us what happened to her on her first day of school. Her teacher told her

> To sit next to Marta, next to her desk, she didn't say at which desk, so I wanted to tell her that I didn't sit there, that I couldn't because she didn't tell me where, and so she yelled at me and said "next to Marta" and I thought that was wrong and I sat down next to Marta, and then she said, "Don't you understand who Marta is", and I did know, but she didn't tell me whether to sit on the left or on the right.

(D) Friendship

Children experience friendship as one of the most important aspects of their biography. It is when they are asked about their friends and what they do together that they speak the most. At these ages, friendship is predominantly valued in quantitative terms: the more friends, the better. Relationships with the other gender range from ignorance and rejection to discovery.

The children's stories reveal four characteristics of their relationship with friends: (a) *Help*: a friend is someone who is willing to help. (b) *Fun*: a friend is someone who is fun to be with. (c) *Trust*: a friend is someone who certain things can be revealed to. (d) *Reciprocity*: a friend is someone who I can treat as I expect to be treated. These four characteristics show an evolution in the childhood concept of friendship from the instrumental relationship of help to the personal relationship considered an end on its own.

Much like in their relationships with their brothers and sisters, conflicts with friends, whether in or out of school, are usually manifestations of the search for self-assertion. The experiences the children recount in their stories are anything but idyllic. Many of these stories tell of teasing, intimidation, bullying, bodily harm and blackmail. Sometimes they involve physical abuse; in other cases, the abuse is more often psychological and affective.

(E) The World of Make-Believe

The world the children imagine when they close their eyes sheds light on their keys to interpretation, their hopes and their current values. In that world, harmony is everywhere, families are together, parents help their children and children help their parents. There, everyone is content, and the only thing that matters is being happy. No one needs to study, because everyone already knows everything. It is a world of nature, full of plants and animals, light shines everywhere and the predominant colour is green.

The world they imagine is largely the counterpart of the aspects the children perceive most negatively in the real world. Patricia, 9 years old, imagines a world *"with houses, instead of sheet metal, they're pretty houses that don't have piles of trash, where everyone is inside eating at a normal kitchen table, not there on the floor, and everyone has a job"*.

We were greatly struck by the fact that a powerful motif in the stories about the world they would like to live in is solitude. The children often wish to be alone in that world. The reason why was told to us by 10-year-old Alba. She said she likes to think that she is alone in her world, *"because I like to see things alone. Because if not, for example, you're thinking one thing and someone else suddenly says: 'look, there's something over there!' and takes away the dream or whatever"*. Stories such as this reveal the search for a more fulfilling experience of one's self, without anyone coming in and telling us what to see.

And from their self, they also discover the other as another self, a subject capable of initiative and decision. Jaime is not sure whether his friends would be in the natural, unpolluted world he imagines, *"because I haven't asked them if they like pollution or not"* (Jaime, age 12). He acknowledges his friends' right to choose and decide for themselves about their own ideal world.

4 Ongoing Research: "Growing Happy"

Proceeding on from our previous experience in exploring children's voices, our last step tries to delve deeper into the way they experience happiness. Many studies on happiness have been carried out in recent years. This kind of research is founded on two ideas: first, that happiness is an attainable aspiration in our lives, and second, that a "good life" depends on more than merely good material living conditions, but finally on concern over social indicators, living standards, childhood policies and welfare policies. From a more pedagogical point of view, what we are trying to answer are the following questions: "What makes children feel happy?" and "How can we use this information for education?"

4.1 Starting Point

A recent report by UNICEF-Innocenti on the living conditions of children in economically advanced nations notes that Spain ranks as one of the countries with the highest child welfare, behind the Netherlands, Sweden, Denmark and Finland, and ahead of the rest of the 21 countries surveyed.[2] Specifically, on the dimension of "subjective well-being", as scientific literature has traditionally called "happiness", Spain is second only to the Netherlands. This data contrasts with other indicators from the same report such as academic achievement on which Spanish children rank low (UNICEF, 2007).

These results suggest that a "hedonic" concept of well-being is not enough to understand the pedagogical meaning of happiness. As Robert F. Dearden (1972) points out,

> The aim of education cannot *simply* be happiness quite without qualification. In education, as in life, there are a number of final ends constitutive of the good of the human being, and on some occasions we may judge some of them properly and rightly to overrule personal happiness, even if for a time the result is that we are less pleased with ourselves or with our lives (p. 111).

Pedagogically, we need to advance to a normative or "eudaimonic" concept of happiness. This is the orientation that has guided our research.

4.2 Fieldwork

As in the previous study, the fieldwork we have just finished was carried out with Spanish primary school children from the 1st to 6th grade. We used two research techniques to elicit answers to the questions raised. For the older group (3rd–6th grade, aged 8–12 years), we designed a questionnaire. For the younger students (1st and 2nd grade, aged 6–8 years), however, we carried out a narrative interview based on the questionnaire and a drawing entitled "your happiest and saddest day". The data was gathered in a sample of 817 children from five primary schools (three public schools and two private state-subsidized schools). As set out in Table 1, a total of 81 children between 6 and 8 years of age were given the interview, and 736 students from 3rd to 6th grade filled out our questionnaire.

---

[2]Components: health (percentage of young people rating their own health no more than "fair" or "poor"); school life (percentage of young people "liking school a lot"); personal well-being (percentage of children rating themselves above the mid-point of a "Life Satisfaction Scale"; percentage of children reporting negatively about personal well-being).

Table 1 Sample characteristics

	Interview and drawing		Questionnaire			
Grade	1	2	3	4	5	6
Age	6–7	7–8	8–9	9–10	10–11	11–12
Number	35	46	170	218	179	169

In order to find out what makes children happy and what they think about happiness, we put children at the centre of our investigation. This perspective is what gives unity to the methodologies employed. It provides the key to not only constructing the questionnaire and the interview but also to interpreting the results. The questions in both the questionnaire and the interviews seek to address five fields involved in the perception children have of their own happiness: (a) self-satisfaction, (b) vital events and everyday situations, (c) aspirations, (d) mastery, and (e) relationships. The following takes a closer look at the content of the questionnaire:

For the first question, we drew the "Stairs of Happiness"[3] in which the child had to place himself or herself on one of the 10 steps.

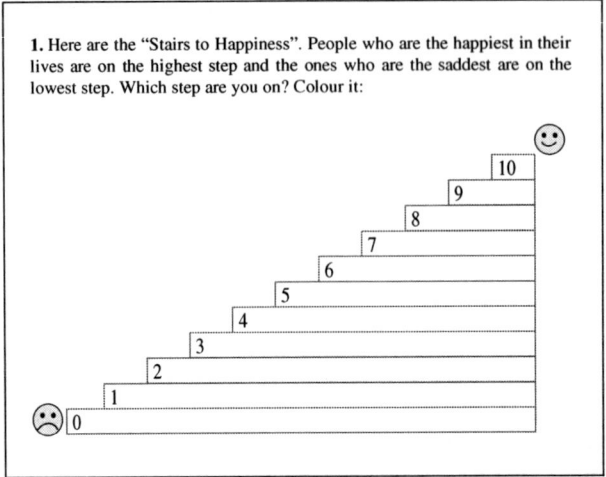

1. Here are the "Stairs to Happiness". People who are the happiest in their lives are on the highest step and the ones who are the saddest are on the lowest step. Which step are you on? Colour it:

After that, we asked children what kind of things made them happy or sad, and what had been the happiest and the saddest day of their life.

2. What kind of things make you happy?	3. What kind of things make you sad?
4. What was the happiest day in your life? What happened on that day?	
5. What wasthe saddest day in your life? What happened on that day?	

---

[3] Based on Cantril's self-anchoring scale.

Then we asked them about their short- and long-term aspirations and what kinds of things they are "good at", or when their families or teachers notice and praise their skills.

6. Do you think you will be happy when you grow up? Why?	
7. What would be your strongest wish?	**8.** What type of things do your teachers praise you for?
9. What type of things do your parents praise you for?	**10.** Write down three things you are very good at.

The final question uses a special technique through pictures. We wanted the children to tell us what they value as an experience of happiness within the various dimensions of their lives. Our focus is on the family, school, playing alone and playing with peers. To the extent that happiness is understandable in terms of action and projection, we have used real photographs to depict each of these areas. The pictures are meant to portray the action of the relevant events in the everyday life of any girl or boy in our country (in this case, a girl called Raquel).

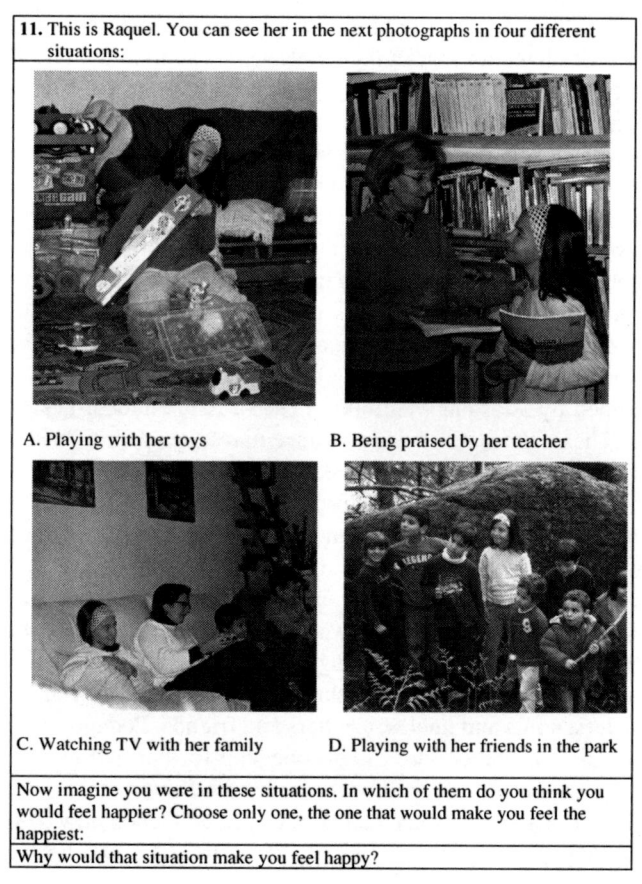

11. This is Raquel. You can see her in the next photographs in four different situations:

A. Playing with her toys   B. Being praised by her teacher

C. Watching TV with her family   D. Playing with her friends in the park

Now imagine you were in these situations. In which of them do you think you would feel happier? Choose only one, the one that would make you feel the happiest:

Why would that situation make you feel happy?

5 Conclusion

Current research on childhood insists on the need to listen to the children's own voices. The line of research being pursued over the last 12 years by the Research Group on Pedagogy of Children's Values has been sensitive to that issue.

The need to hear the children's voices may be justified from three perspectives: epistemological, ethical and pedagogical. From an epistemological point of view, today we realize that knowledge of childhood experience cannot be obtained simply by inference—that is to say, based on the meaning we adults give to that experience. Rather, it necessitates listening to the children's own voices. Ethically, we acknowledge that children have rights, and not just rights to protection, but also the right to express themselves and be heard on matters concerning them. Finally, from a pedagogical perspective, there is no question today of the need to consider children as agents of their own learning process, instead of as mere containers of the intentions we adults bestow on them. It is also generally agreed that an essential element of the educational task is to know the learner, to know how to put oneself in that learner's shoes, to capture life from that learner and use that knowledge to help him or her to follow his or her own path.

The biographical research with children we have presented here has allowed us to find a number of elements specifying what we have called the childhood ethical experience of being in the world. To anyone who works in the field of childhood education, these results may give them better knowledge of the children's own subjective experience and how they experience their reality. Nevertheless, from a pedagogical point of view, we cannot stop here. We must go one step further, and in light of our results, ask about the meaning itself of narrative experience in education.

The narrative approach largely reflects an influx of epistemological postmodernism and notions such as intertextuality in which the subject, deprived of a constitutive core, dissolves into a series of narratives, and in which there is no place for pedagogic intentionality. Late twentieth century philosophy, however, provides us with other ways of understanding the narrative meaning of identity, such as the ones developed by Alasdair MacIntyre (1981), Paul Ricoeur (1990) or Charles Taylor (1992). These alternative views restore narrative identity within normative horizons, and justify the possibility of reading our stories in terms of pedagogic effects. Seen in these terms, the most prominent result we have achieved in our research is probably that discovery of oneself and the other as subjects that runs through the narratives.

That other, who, as Ricoeur would say, is discovered on the edges of the narrative experience, must be understood here in two different ways: first, the other as distinct from me. In the children's stories, narrating is telling the story of a bond with certain communities of belonging, starting with the ones closest by. These are their parents, brothers and sisters, aunts and uncles, teachers and friends. Pedagogical intervention then resides in teaching the children to go one step further and use these domains of relationships to open up not only to the nearest other or others, but also to the other far away. Narrative experience can help us see and teach how to see any other as another biography, with her or his own affects, troubles and hopes; as another unique being whose life spreads out in everyday aspirations. Thus, in this first sense, the pedagogical potentiality—and the limitation—of narrative experience must be situated in its ability to open us up to the other as another self.

However, biographical experience also opens me up to the other that I am and can be, because my narrating means being able to become an object of my own story-telling. This, then, is an effect that complements the previous one. If previously the pedagogical intention was to learn to see the other as a self, it now becomes to learn to see oneself as an other, as the other yet to be, the experience of possibility and deficit that, ever since Socratic pedagogy, constitutes the driving force of education.

References

Bruner, J. (1996). *Realidad mental y mundos posibles*. Barcelona: Gedisa.

Dearden, R. F. (1972). Happiness and education. In R. F. Dearden, P.H. Hirst, & R. S. Peters (Eds.), *Education and the development of reason* (pp. 95–111). London: Routledge and Kegan Paul.

Gil, F., & Jover, G. (1998). La experiencia de los derechos humanos en contextos de aprendizaje escolar: una investigación a través de las nuevas tecnologías. *Revista Española de Pedagogía, 211*, 561–585.

Gil, F., & Jover, G. (2000). Las tendencias narrativas en pedagogía y la aproximación biográfica al mundo infantil. *Enrahonar, 31*, 107–122.

Gil, F., & Jover, G. (2003). La contribución de la educación ética y política en la formación del ciudadano. *Revista de Educación. Special issue, 1*, 109–129.

Gil, F., Jover, G., & Reyero, D. (2003). La educación moral ante las guerras y los conflictos. *Teoría de la Educación. Revista Interuniversitaria, 15*, 161–183.

Gil, F., Jover, G., & Reyero, D. (2006). La educación de la sensibilidad solidaria desde la reconstrucción de la memoria lúdica. *Teoría de la Educación. Revista Interuniversitaria, 18*, 153–174.

Jover, G. (2001). What does the right to education mean? A look at an international debate from legal, ethical, and pedagogical points of view. *Studies in Philosophy and Education, 20*(3), 213–223.

Jover, G., & Reyero, D. (2000). Images of the other in childhood: Researching the limits of cultural diversity in education from the standpoint of new anthropological methodologies. *Encounters on Education, 1*, 125–152.

MacIntyre, A. (1981). *After virtue*. Notre Dame: University of Notre Dame Press.

Ricoeur, P. (1990). *Soi-même comme un autre*. Paris: Editions du Seuil.

Taylor, C. (1992). *Sources of the self*. Cambridge: Cambridge University Press.

UNICEF. (2007). *Child poverty in perspective: An overview of child well-being in rich countries*. Florence: UNICEF Innocenti Research Centre.

Researching Identities, Difference, Subjectivities and Social Relations in Childhood Within Multi-ethnic Infant and Primary School Settings

Cecile Wright

1 Introduction

How society rids itself of such attitudes is not something which we can prescribe, except to stress the need for education and example at the youngest age, and an overall attitude of 'Zero tolerance' of racism within our society.

(Report of the Stephen Lawrence Inquiry (Macpherson, 1999) para. 7.42)

What kind of school do we want to learn in? We want a school where ALL pupils LOOK OUT FOR EACH OTHER.

('Listening: Pupils' voices, experiences and advice', from Preventing and Addressing Racism in Schools, Ealing Council 2003 in the UK)

The increasing diversity, in Britain and other countries, means that children interact with different cultures, languages, faiths and traditions on a regular basis

'A Good Childhood': Searching for Values in a Competitive Age (2009: 20), The Children Society, Penguin

The above quotations ostensively offer commentary on aspects of childhood, particularly in relation to the late twentieth and the beginning of the twenty-first century. They highlight themes concerning race and racism, the centrality of embracing difference, diversity and creating an environment for all children to develop positive attitudes about themselves. They also posit the role of social institutions such as education in inculcating these values during the period of childhood. Interestingly, against this background, however, there is the expressed ideal of creating the environment for all children to develop positive attitudes about themselves and other people unlike themselves, as well as to have the opportunity to learn with, from and about each other in multicultural settings. In this, education has played a rather

C. Wright (✉)
School of Social Sciences, Nottingham Trent University, Nottingham,
Nottinghamshire NG1 4BU, UK
e-mail: cecile.wright@ntu.ac.uk

S. Andresen et al. (eds.), *Children and the Good Life*, Children's Well-Being: Indicators and Research 4, DOI 10.1007/978-90-481-9219-9_10,
© Springer Science+Business Media B.V. 2010

ambivalent role. Historically, within the United Kingdom, the presence of black[1] and minority ethnic (BME) pupils within the education system has been framed within a discourse of being problematic, in particular, of their potentially negative impact on schools and other (i.e. White) pupils as a result of their 'alien demands and identities'. Archer/Francis (2007: 1) argue that although, within the policy domain, 'approaches to "race" have changed over the years, the pathologisation of minority ethnic pupils within education policy remains an issue today—although debates have taken a more subtle and complex form'.

This chapter is about young children's educational experience. It is set in the United Kingdom (UK), and is concerned with exploring how 'race'/racism enters young children's social world and shapes identities, subjectivity, social relations and agency within the context of schooling.

Research conducted in the fields of sociology and the sociology of education has shed valuable light on the ways in which older children construct racialised identities (e.g. Alexander, 1996; Back, 1996; Dwyer, 2000), and, specifically, it has examined black and minority ethnic young people's experiences of racialised identities within the context of education or schooling (Alexander, 1996; Archer, 2003; Back, 1996; Dwyer, 2000; Mirza, 1992; Sewell, 1987; Wright, 1987; Wright, Standen, & Patel, 2010). Within the literature, with the exception of a few studies (e.g. Connolly, 1998; Wright, 1992), we find a distinct lack of attention being paid to younger black and minority ethnic children's own experiences and concerns. It is precisely this tendency to ignore the subjective experiences and concerns of young children, particularly in relation to 'race'/ethnicity, the significance of 'race' in the development of young children's identities, and how it informs their social world that pervaded my study into children's lives in the 1990s. This study examined the experiences of young children of Asian and African-Caribbean backgrounds in nursery/infant and middle school settings in the UK and their negotiation of race/racism in their relations with other children.

The chapter is concerned with examining young children's social world within the context of schooling, particularly in relation to diversity and difference. In particular, it raises the matter of the extent to which their experiences of schooling and their emerging social identities and subjectivity can be understood while recognising the importance they give to the exploration, negotiation and development of racialised discourses in their day-to-day lives. It draws on a study performing a detailed exploration of young children's social world through an in-depth study of 3–13-year-old children in several English multiethnic, inner-city nursery, primary and middle schools in the 1990s. It was particularly concerned with understanding the complex ways in which 'race'/racism intervenes in young children's lives and comes to shape their identities. It was recognised that while these processes are clearly evident among the young children's peer-group cultures, they can only be understood by tracing their origins to social organisations of the school and the

---

[1] 'Black' refers to people who have at least one parent of African Caribbean descent. 'South Asian' refers to people who have descended from India, Pakistan or Bangladesh. It is recognised that such a definition is problematic in that it draws together people with very different ethnic, religious and/or national identities.

community. Indeed, as Bronfenbrenner (1979) emphasised, the notion that development is influenced by human interactions within specific settings, the relationship between these settings and the larger context within which these settings are situated further informs my approach. Of course, the school is one of the major settings in which the child acts out the complex and simple interactions of individuals with others, and where the actions and reactions between participants are significant (Upton & Cooper, 1991).

2 The Theorising of 'Whiteness', 'Race'/Ethnicity

The results reported here come from an empirical study aimed at understanding the nature of racism in young children's lives and the ways in which it comes to influence their identities. The study also reveals the processes and practices in the production and reproduction of racialised discourses among children and draws on 'whiteness studies' and theorising of 'race'/ethnicity.

There is a variety of ways of conceptualising terms such as 'white' and 'whiteness' (see Dyer, 1997; Frankenberg, 1993; Levine-Rasky, 2002). Here, 'white' is taken to mean the racially dominant group of European descent (see Leonardo, 2004). 'Whiteness' is a process involving the acquisition of social dominance by whites (e.g. Dyer, 1997). It is not necessarily simply an issue of white bodies. 'Whiteness' is socially constructed to such an extent that it is taken for granted as the norm (Frankenberg, 1993). One possible consequence of this is that racialised others ('non-whites') can only be known in relation to 'whiteness' (Bonnett, 1997). Whiteness gains much of its power by being taken as the norm. It is argued that since 'whiteness' is taken for granted and taken as the norm, non-white identities become marginal and are seen as 'inferior' (e.g. Levine-Rasky, 2002). So whiteness gains a 'supremacy' culturally and biologically such that racialised others (non-whites) are seen to lack the qualities ascribed to whites. Within the context of education or schooling, Leonardo (2004) states '. . .. black and ethnic minority students' benefit from schooling that reveals to them the implications of whiteness, because they have to understand the daily vicissitudes of white discourses and be able to deal with them. That is, in order to confront/respond to whiteness, they have to be familiar with it. In the process, they realise that their ethnicity is relational to whiteness's claim of colour-blindness and both are burst asunder in the process. Thus, the goal is for BME students to engage whiteness while simultaneously working to dismantle it. Whereas, white students benefit from neo-abolitionism because they come to terms with the daily fears associated with the upkeep of whiteness. In so far as whiteness is a performance (Giroux, 1997), white students possess a vulnerable persona always an inch away from being exposed as bogus. The daily white performance is dependent on the assertion of a false world built on rickety premises' (p. 119).

In addition to the above discussion of 'whiteness' as a 'racial discourse', as an identity and as a signifier of privilege, it is also pertinent to be mindful of theorising 'race'/ethnicity. For instance, the work of Stuart Hall (e.g. 1992) has made an important contribution by disrupting fixed notions of race, ethnicity, culture and

racism. In particular, 'traditional' and commonsense notions about race as a biological phenomenon have been challenged (Miles, 1989). Instead, it has been argued
that race is an ideological, not a scientific, construct (denoted as 'race'), and attention has been drawn to the ways in which 'race' is constituted, challenged and
reformed through multiple discourses across time and space. 'Race' is thus unsta-
ble and 'constantly being transformed by political struggle'. However, as Hall's
work also reminds us, 'race' is a fiction that has very 'real' material and symbolic
consequences (e.g. Hall, 1992, p. 226). In accordance with the retheorisation of
ethnicity, 'race' and identity, it has been argued that it is not possible to speak of
any singular or coherent notion of 'racism' either. Rather, critical sociological and
psychological thinking has moved towards understanding multiple racisms, which
include subtle and complex articulations and formations that are not just attitudinal, interpersonal or behavioural, but can also be unwittingly structurally enacted
via interpersonal communication as well as by individuals or groups. In this vein,
while identity can be viewed as internal, personally led and psychologically driven,
it is recognised that it has to be located within broader societal constructions and
limitations—for example, around social categories of 'youth', 'race'/ethnicity, gender, social class/socioeconomic status, and so on, as well as within social groupings
such as nations, communities or families.

The data reported here highlights influences on young children's construction of
racialised identities. It reflects on the power of whiteness to shape the children's
everyday experiences. Moreover, the data draws attention to the variety of contexts (e.g. classrooms, wider school localities) within which children were located
and how, within each, discourses on 'race' came to be appropriated, reworked and
reproduced in a diverse number of ways. Each of these aspects is explored below.

3 Negotiating Differences in Developing a Racialised Self

Reading ethnographic studies on 'race', the early years and schooling, you could
be forgiven for reaching the conclusion that an aspect of the 'primary ideology' is
a form of pedagogic folklore which, inter alia, views childhood as an age of innocence. Regarding issues of 'race and ethnicity', the popular belief still exists among
teachers that young children are 'colour-blind'. Moreover, primary teachers assume
that young children, whilst capable of unacceptable behaviour, remain free from
the malign influences of individual racism. However, the following verbal accounts
from a nursery classroom encounter highlight how young children reflected their
awareness of racial and ethnic differences in conversation with both teachers/carers
and peers, and attributed value to these differences. For example, the discussion
between Charlene, a 3-year-old black girl (of African-Caribbean background), and
Tina, a 4-year-old white girl during creative play at Castle School[2] illustrates this
perfectly.

---

[2]The names of schools are pseudonyms.

Charlene: (Cuddling a black doll) This is my baby.

Tina: I don't like it, it's funny. I like this one (holding a white doll), it's my favourite. I don't like this one (pointing at the black doll). Because you see I like Sarah, and I like white. You're my best friend though, you're brown.

Charlene: I don't like that one (pointing to the white doll).

Tina: You're brown aren't you?

Charlene: I'm not brown, I'm black.

Tina: You're brown, but I'm white.

Charlene: No I'm not, I'm black and baby's black.

Tina: They call us white, my mummy calls me white, and you know my mummy calls you brown. When you come to visit if you want... She'll say 'hello brown person'. I like brown not black. Michael Jackson was brown, he went a bit white.

It could be argued that it is through these discourses on racial difference that some children come to develop their sense of identity. What is interesting from the conversation is Tina's desire not to offend, and her struggle to locate Charlene with the construction of blackness. The dynamics underlying this unease related to the desire to maintain their friendship. Also of interest is the appropriation from popular culture by citing Michael Jackson to support her argument about the 'fuzziness of identity'. Moreover, arising from the children's discussion of difference is not just acknowledgement of their 'difference', but rather the more difficult question of the kind of difference that is acknowledged and engaged.

4 'Othering' Difference

This theme is concerned with exploring the extent to which children develop their own identities in opposition to the others. Classroom observations in the study also suggest that children at this early age were showing a preference for members of their own racial/ethnic group and a desire to mix and play with them rather than with others. This 'own-group' preference did on occasion reflect antipathy towards children of another skin colour or cultural groups. The children's preference for members of their own racial/ethnic group is corroborated by an African Caribbean Child Care Assistant at Bridgeway School:

The white children, particularly a set of white children, even though they related to me and Sharan (Asian Carer) all right, they won't play with anybody else, when I say with anybody else I mean black or Asian children. There are a couple of black children that won't play with Asian children, but they won't play with white children either. I've noticed that the Asian children play very well and they play well amongst themselves and alongside each other, but they don't mix themselves as well... But I think there is an attitude in the school that makes the Asian children feel negative about themselves as well.

A significant number of boys and girls within the school seemed to develop their own identities in opposition to children, particularly Asian children. For instance, at this early age, white children tended to be extremely negative towards the Asian children both in their attitudes and behaviour. They often refused to play with them and frequently subjected them to threatening behaviour, name calling and hitting. An example of this theme is explored in the following incident at Bridgeway

School. A group of four white boys (aged 3–4 years) were collaboratively building a tower block out of building blocks. An Asian boy walked over with the
thought of participating. Two of the boys were heard to say vehemently 'No Paki,
no Paki'. Another boy pushed the Asian boy aggressively. The Asian boy wandered
off looking dejected.

The nursery teachers/carers were also aware of similar incidents of this nature.
As an African-Caribbean carer at Bridgeway School pointed out,

> Peter... [the] blond headed boy, I notice that he used to go up to the Asian children in a
> really threatening way, just threatening behaviour. He wouldn't say anything. If the Asian
> children had anything he would take it off them. They'd leave something if they were
> playing with it. He would look at them and they would drop it.

In the classroom, white children engaged in persistent racist name calling, teasing, jostling, intimidation, rejection and the occasional physical assault on black and
ethnic minority children. Aspects of this behaviour are illustrated in the following
incident from Adelle School. I was in a classroom observing and working with a
group of six white 6-year-olds on English language and number tasks. Taseem (an
Asian girl) came over to the group and, with a rather desperate look on her face,
asked me to help her.

> Taseem: Miss Cecile, can you help me do times by?

Taseem was working on a multiplication exercise which she did not fully understand. The 10 sums she had completed for this exercise had been marked as incorrect
by the teacher, and she had been asked to do the exercise again. I spent some minutes
explaining the exercise to Taseem. The children in the group were very resentful of
the fact that I had switched my attention from them to Taseem and also that she had
joined the group.

> CW: (After having finished explaining the exercise) Taseem, do you understand how 'times
>   by' works?
> Jane (a white girl): No, she won't understand, she's a Paki.
> Taseem is very upset by this comment and is on the verge of tears.
> CW: (to Jane) What do you mean?
> Jane: Because she's a Paki.
>   The other children in the group were sniggering.
> CW: And why should she not understand multiplications because she's Pakistani?
> Jane: Because she's not one of us and she's not our culture.
>   Michael (a white boy): She's a Paki! (laughs).
> CW: What is our culture?
> Jane: England.
> CW: She is in England, she lives in England.
> Jane: Yeah, but she comes from Pakistan.
> Alice (a white girl): Yeah, Pakistani, she was born in Pakistan she means.
> Taseem: (dejected but not protesting) I wasn't. I was born here.
> Jane: She couldn't understand, that's what I think because she's a Paki
> Other children: (to Taseem) Where were you born?
> CW: Yes, just because she speaks 'Pakistani' it does not mean that she can't understand
>   how to multiply.

Jane: Because when I say something, she doesn't know what I say. And when assembly they were doing a Paki dance.

CW: Taseem was born in England, her parents are from Pakistan, but she was born in England.

Taseem: My parents are here.

The researcher continues to assist Taseem with her number work. The other children become increasingly resentful.

Jane: (sharply) Will you help me now?

Some of the children take to taunting and name calling Taseem. However, sensing my disapproval of their behaviour, they adopt a strategy of name calling by sounding out the letters.

Jane: P-A-K-E, P-A-K-E!

Alice: (quietly spoken) She's a Paki!

CW: What does P-A-K-E mean?

Jane: (with a mischievous grin, whispering) She's a Paki!

Taseem: (visibly distraught) Miss, I want to go out and play.

Echoing of P-A-K-E from the other children.

Alice: She's a Paki, that's what it means.

This encounter not only highlights that some South Asian children have been adversely positioned within some children's racist discourses, but also shows that some of the children were struggling with the appropriateness of the racist term 'Paki'. On recognising my displeasure with their remarks, they endeavoured to disguise their intent. Underlying many of these discourses was the construction of Asian children as the 'other': as inferior and 'alien'. It could be argued that this highlights the reproduction of wider societal discourses within the field of peer relations. Further, the teachers, with only a few exceptions, mentioned the extent to which this construction of Asian children as the 'other' was prevalent in relation in the field of peer groups. Indeed, the white children's attitude and behaviour towards the Asian children was a concern for the majority of teachers. A teacher at Adelle School explained,

> The Asian children are getting so picked on, it's awful. In the playground the Asian girls never leave the teacher's side. One little girl last week, they [white children] never left her alone, she was really frightened. I mean she really did need protection... but we can't stand next to her all the time. Every time I looked, somebody was at her.

One strategy for avoiding expressions of racial intolerance was to separate children of different ethnic groups. The following teacher's comment was typical of many that were expressed to me:

> I have to think very carefully when I select children to work together because, more often than not, white children will refuse to sit next to or work with a Pakistani. You have to bear this in mind so as to avoid any nastiness.

This comment can be seen as an indication that racism is 'taken for granted' rather than something to be explored or challenged. Moreover, the young white children's narrative illustrates how non-white identities become marginal and are seen as 'inferior'. Also, the children's discourse accords with Frankenberg's (1993, p. 1) discussion of how the social construction of whiteness outlines 'linked dimensions' which give shape and meaning to whiteness and race privilege—also as being a standpoint 'from which white people look at ourselves, at others and at society' and lastly as a 'set of cultural practices'. Additionally, the children's narratives reveal the processes of 'being and becoming' a raced (and gendered) subject of educational (or schooling) discourse.

5 Conclusion and Implications

This chapter is concerned with the educational experience of young children and how they negotiate race/racism in their relations with other children. It fills a gap in research by examining the experiences of young children and the significance of 'race' in the development of their identities.

It also addresses the notion of 'whiteness' and how it is taken as a norm. The idea that young children are 'colour blind' is also tackled. Classroom observations reveal clear processes of 'othering' on the basis of 'race' both in the classroom and in play. Racist name calling is common and enhances the construction of Asian children as 'other'. More generally, the chapter asks the still necessary and fundamental questions regarding research on identities, difference, subjectivities and social relations in childhood. Some of these include issues relating to

1. The social competence of children as young as 3, 4 and 6 in reflecting upon and intervening in their social world
2. The skill with which some children are able to actively appropriate, rework and reproduce discourses on 'race', difference and diversity in quite complex ways
3. How emphasis on the agency of young children has helped bring into focus what has been termed their 'decentred selves'
4. The extent to which children's identities are therefore not simply determined by their age but also by their gender, ethnicity, class and so forth
5. How these all come together within specific contexts to provide the background against which children develop their sense of identity
6. More fundamentally, it questions the appropriateness of making assumptions about children's cognitive ability or their level of awareness on matters of 'race' simply by their age
7. Drawing attention to the ability of children to acquire a relatively sophisticated and active understanding of their social worlds
8. Demonstrating the ability to research the subjectivities of young children, but also drawing attention to the particular methods that appear to be most suitable (of course not without issues-researcher effects)
9. The essential and contingent nature of the young children's racialised identities. It draws attention to the variety of contexts within which children are located and how, within each context, discourses on 'race' come to be appropriated, reworked and reproduced in a diverse number of ways.

References

Alexander, C. (1996). *The art of being black: The creation of black British youth identities*. Oxford: Oxford University Press.

Archer, L. (2003). *'Race', Masculinity and Schooling: Muslim boys and Education*. Buckingham: Open University Press.

Archer, L., & Francis, B. (2007). *Understanding minority ethnic achievement: 'Race', gender, class and 'success'*. London: Routledge.

Back, L. (1996). *New ethnicities and urban culture: Racism and multiculture in young lives*. London: UCL Press.

Bonnett, A. (1997). Constructions of whiteness in European and American anti-racism. In P. Webner & T. Modood (Eds.), *Debating cultural hybridity: Multi-cultural identities and the politics of anti-racism* (pp. 173–180). London: Zed Books.

Bronfenbrenner, U. (1979). *The ecology of human development: Experiments by nature and design*. Cambridge, MA: Harvard University Press.

Connolly, P. (1998). *Racism, gender identities and young children*. London: Routledge.

Dwyer, C. (2000). Negotiating diasporic identities: Young British south Asian Muslim women. *Women's Studies International Forum, 23*(4), 475–486.

Dyer, R. (1997). *White*. London: Routledge.

Frankenberg, R. (Ed.). (1993). *White women, race matters: The social organization of whiteness*. Minneapolis, MI: University of Minnesota Press.

Giroux, H. (1997). Rewriting the discourse of racial identity: Towards a pedagogy and politics of whiteness. *Harvard Educational Review, 67*, 285–320.

Hall, S. (1992). New ethnicities. In J. Donald & A. Rattansi (Eds.), *'Race', culture and difference* (pp. 252–259). London: Sage.

Leonardo, Z. (2004). The souls of white folk: Critical pedagogy, whiteness studies and globalization discourse. In G. Ladson-Billings & D. Gillborn (Eds.), *The Routledge falmer reader in multicultural education*. London: Routledge Falmer.

Levine-Rasky, C. (2002). *Working through whiteness: International perspectives*. Albany, NY: State University of New York Press.

Macpherson, W. (1999). *The Stephen Lawrence inquiry: Report of a inquiry by Sir William Macpherson of Clancy*. London: The Stationery Office.

Miles, R. (1989). *Racism*. London: Routledge.

Mirza, H. (1992). *Young, female and black*. London: Routledge.

Sewell, T. (1987). *Black masculinities and schooling: How black boys survive modern schooling*. Stoke-on-Trent: Trentham Books.

Upton, G., & Cooper, P. (1991). A new perspective on behaviour problems in school: The ecosystemic approach. *Maladjustment and Therapeutic Education, 8*(1), 3–18.

Wright, C. (1987). Black students – White teachers. In B. Troyna (Ed.), *Racial inequality in education* (pp. 109–126). London: Allen and Unwin.

Wright, C. (1992). *'Race relations' in the primary school*. London: David Fulton Publishers.

Wright, C., Standen, P., & Patel, T. (2010). *Black youth matters: Transitions from school to success*. New York: Routledge.

Childhood Studies in Turkey

Akile Gürsoy

1 Introduction

The paradox is the singularity of each childhood against the universality of childhood itself (Fernea, 2002, p. 2).

An overview commentary on the state of childhood studies in Turkey means talking about social change and history. Each culture is embedded with particular modes of relating to and rearing children. The socialization and education of children has been a predominant occupation of all cultures. The concept of childhood also contains in itself the concept of adulthood. It has been noted that becoming an adult member of one's society means more than merely learning its skills, however difficult these may be. An adult must also be given recognition by the remainder of society: Adulthood is defined socially and not in terms of physical or psychological maturity alone. Especially today, no culture can stand alone. Rather, social groups constantly redefine themselves in relation to contact with other cultures. As an expression of the approach of the Council on Intercultural Relations in the United States, Margaret Mead asked in 1941, "What effects has the mingling of peoples— of different races, different religions, different levels of cultural complexity—had upon our concept of education?" (1941/1970, p. 2). One may add to this, what has changed in our understanding of childhood?

Since the appearance of Philippe Aries' classic work *Centuries of Childhood* (1962), much scholarly attention has been devoted to the conceptualization and study of childhood by different disciplines including psychology, psychiatry, education, social work, sociology, anthropology, history and legal studies. Children have been the focus of research from a variety of perspectives. However, as Perrig-Chiello (2009) has noted,

Even though significant advances in European research and social reporting on childhood and youth have been observed in the last two decades, there is still a

A. Gürsoy (✉)
Faculty of Arts and Sciences, Yeditepe University, 81120 Kayışdağı, Istanbul, Turkey
e-mail: akile@yeditepe.edu.tr

S. Andresen et al. (eds.), *Children and the Good Life*, Children's Well-Being: Indicators and Research 4, DOI 10.1007/978-90-481-9219-9_11,
© Springer Science+Business Media B.V. 2010

great need for action due to the ongoing demographic and societal changes, which have a direct and far-reaching impact on the lives of children and adolescents and their families (p. 3).

2 Childhood in the Early Years of the Republic of Turkey

In the early years of the Republic of Turkey, childhood and children were conceptualized by the governing elite as the core of the life force and sustainability of the newly founded state. At the turn of the century, the last years of the Ottoman Empire were characterized by extremely poor public health. Estimates indicate about one-half of the population of Anatolia was inflicted with malaria. In some villages in the south, about 70% of the population was estimated to be suffering from the disease. In a population of about 13 million, about one million were said to have tuberculosis. Due to years of continued wars and their cumulative effects, (the Crimean war, the Balkan wars, the wars in Yemen and Palestine, World War I), the number of handicapped people was very high. About one-fifth of the households had no adult male. Life expectancy was 35 years (Gürsoy, 1998, p. 42; Şehsuvaroğlu, 1984, p. 170).

Maternal and child mortality rates were extremely high as well. It is estimated that about one out of three children died before reaching their fifth year. In fact, it is known that Atatürk and his circle of friends feared that the population of Turkey would diminish and disappear the way some native populations had lost their effectiveness in the Americas. To ensure the continuity of the population, pronatalist policies were adopted. Childbirth was encouraged and measures taken to increase the well-being of children. For example, competitions were organized to award prizes for chubby and robust babies and children. Mothers with high numbers of healthy children were praised and awarded. Motherhood was exalted. It is noteworthy that during these years, Germany was regarded as a positive role model for childrearing practices for disciplined motherhood.[1]

Following the War of Independence, the Republic of Turkey rose on the ruins of the Ottoman Empire. The 23rd of April, 1920 is the day the Turkish National Assembly was opened. Initially, this date was celebrated as the day of "National Sovereignty". As a reflection on the importance attributed to children and childhood, Atatürk later honoured children, and, in 1935, the day became celebrated as "National Sovereignty and Children's Day". Through the generations, this has become an official tradition. This day is instituted as a gift to the children of Turkey. On this day, children throughout the country sit in the seats of high-ranking officials like the head of parliament or the prime minister; in cities and towns, of the mayor; and in schools, in the office of the principal. Children give press interviews and declare what they would do if they held that rank and responsibility. The following

---

[1] In later years, the American model of childrearing practices, in particular Dr. Spock's methods became influential in Turkey.

day is a holiday for primary school students. Even though for just one day, the older generations are invited to realize that in the coming future, it will be today's children who will hold these positions. It is also a symbolic handing down of power to children.

3 Children and Gender in Numbers in Turkey

Today, contrary to the fears of the early Republican era, the population of the country has reached over 70 million (see Table 1), and it is issues of life quality rather than survival that dominate the discourse on the public health of children. In 2008, Turkey had about 19 million children (about 25% of the population) under the age of 15, and about 25 million children under the age of 19. Furthermore, there are more than 4.5 million citizens or former citizens of Turkey living in Europe (Küçükcan/Veyis 2009, p. 1). This migrant population has a relatively higher fertility rate compared with that of the citizens of the countries they inhabit.

The fertility rate in Turkey has declined continually, and is presently 2.16, a rate almost equal to the minimum replacement level of 2.10. The total fertility rate in rural areas is 2.68 compared to 2.00 in urban areas. It varies according to different regions of Turkey, being lowest in western Turkey (1.73) and highest in eastern Turkey (3.27). There is also significant variation according to the level of income

Table 1 Population of Turkey by age and sex (31/12/2008)

Age group	Total	Male	Female	Total age group as % of total pop.
0–4	5,258,988	3,082,338	2,915,020	7.35
5–9	6,318,132	3,242,581	3,075,551	8.83
10–14	6,472,197	3,322,041	3,150,156	9.05
15–19	6,185,104	3,171,917	3,013,187	8.64
20–24	6,256,558	3,187,625	3,068,993	8.75
25–29	6,518,837	3,300,291	3,218,546	9.11
30–34	5,810,107	2,939,518	2,870,589	8.12
35–39	5,330,484	2,680,941	2,649,543	7.45
40–44	4,740,250	2,397,706	2,342,544	6.63
45–49	4,284,175	2,153,427	2,130,748	5.90
50–54	3,643,173	1,824,582	1,818,591	5.09
55–59	2,878,104	1,423,445	1,454,659	4.02
60–64	2,188,298	1,035,261	1,153,037	3.05
65–69	1,701,384	783,680	917,704	2.38
70–74	1,274,681	575,433	699,248	1.78
75–79	1,110,782	492,226	618,556	1.55
80–84	571,179	213,336	357,843	0.80
85–89	175,221	59,076	116,145	0.25
90+	60,176	15,730	44,446	0.08
Total	71,517,100	35,901,154	35,615,946	100

Note: Turkish Bureau of Statistics (TÜİK).

and the education of women: Those with the lowest income have the highest fertility rate (3.39), and those with the highest income have the lowest fertility rate (2.16) (Hacettepe University Institute of Population Studies, 2009, p. 62). The desired ideal number of children expressed by women in Turkey varies on average between 2 and 3 children. Women in the west, women with more education and higher economic status express a lower ideal number of children.

One intriguing issue holds true the world over. In all societies, with the exception of the population over 60, the number of males exceeds the number of females. Is this due to a lack of registration and an indication of missing records? Or does it mean that the survival rates of men are higher than those of women? It is known that new technology makes it possible to determine the sex of the unborn baby, and in traditional societies with a strong preference for sons, abortions may be performed in cases when the family wants to have a baby son and not a baby daughter.

Like the tip of an iceberg, these figures showing higher numbers of boys and men can be very revealing about gender discrimination among boys and girls. More research on this issue is needed the world over.

4 Relationship Between the State and Children

Since its formation, the Republic of Turkey has accepted three constitutions in 1924, 1961 and 1982. All have recognized and emphasized the existence and well-being of the child. The Turkish Constitution (*Anayasa*), which forms the underlying structure of all Turkish laws, mentions children (*çocuk*) directly a number of times; and numerous articles are directly or indirectly aimed at regulating viewpoints related to issues concerning childhood. In the Constitution, children are also referred to as *yetim* (orphans) (Article 66) and as *küçükler* (the small ones) (Article 50). Article 66 shapes the official identity of children born as citizens of Turkey; Article 42 delineates the rights of the child to education; Article 24 guarantees freedom of faith and religion and gives parents the right to give their children appropriate religious education; Article 25 says everyone (*herkes*) has freedom of expression and this includes children; Article 41 states that families in need, mothers and children in particular, are under the protection of the state. Article 62 refers to Turkish citizens working in other countries, and is directly involved in securing the education of the children of workers in foreign countries.[2]

The Turkish Ministry of Social Work and Institution of Child Protection, *Başbakanlık Sosyal Hizmetler ve Çocuk Esirgeme Kurumu*, is the sole officially recognized institution that takes care of orphaned and abandoned children. Children whose parents have died or are unable to give them care are institutionalized and

---

[2]Article 62 states, "The state takes the necessary precautions for securing the family union, the education of the children, the cultural needs and social security; securing the bonds with the mother country of Turkish citizens working in foreign countries, and takes the necessary precautions for helping them when returning home".

raised in this state institution. The adoption laws of the country prohibit the adoption of Turkish children by non-Turkish citizens, or the deportation of orphaned children out of the country.

Even when a child has parents, given the right conditions, the state can always intervene and decide over the fate of the child. The state can choose to get involved and intervene in individual lives in many ways, especially in cases that acquire symbolic importance for state identity. In fact, in the world of nation states, most states have paramount control over individuals.

For example, in January 1996, Turkey and Great Britain experienced much publicized diplomatic confrontation when Musa (19) and Sarah (13) underwent an Islamic marriage in eastern Turkey. Great Britain asked that Sarah, being underage, be sent back. Turkey replied that she was free to return, but that she could not be forced to leave the country. The media reported that 30,000 signatures had been collected from people in Turkey, mostly advocates of an Islamic revivalist party, calling for Sarah to stay in Turkey. Controversies abounded. Both states however united in demonstrating that ultimately children belonged to them and not to their families. Great Britain threatened to take away the parental rights of Sarah's parents who were found guilty of sending their underage daughter into marriage, particularly since this involved a cross-cultural journey. Musa, on the other hand was put in prison by Turkish law for abducting and keeping an underage person (see Gürsoy, 1996a, b).

5 Childhood Studies in Turkey

Presently, there are no comprehensive interdisciplinary academic programmes on childhood in Turkey, similar to programmes on women's studies, urban studies or migration studies. However, a number of research centres exist, mostly to monitor the physical health of children and children's rights in general. Among the most noteworthy is the International Children's Centre based in Bilkent University in Ankara and Istanbul University Çapa Centre for Child Health. Of course, in the more than 100 universities across the country, there are numerous departments of paediatrics, sociology, psychology, and literature as well as individual researchers focusing on children. There is a prolific amount of civil society initiatives, and numerous associations concerned with children. The majority of these focus on special problems encountered in childhood.[3] The Turkish General Directorate of

---

[3] To give a few examples of associations focusing on children, one can cite AÇEV (Mother—Child Education Foundation); Çağdaş Yaşamı Destekleme Derneği (ÇYDD) (Association for the Support of Contemporary Life); Çocuk Vakfı (Children's Foundation); Çocuk ve Bilgi Güvenliği Derneği (Association for Children and Safety of Information)—for the prevention of child abuse; Özel Eğitim Gerektiren Çocuk Hakları Derneği (Association for Child Rights of Children Who Need Special Education); Türkiye Eğitim Gönüllüleri Vakfı (TEGV) (Foundation for Education Volunteers); Türkiye Sokak Çocukları Derneği (Turkish Street Children Association); Umut Çocukları Derneği (Association for Hope Children); Üstün Zekalı ve Yetenekli Çocuklar Derneği (ÜZYEÇDE) (Association for Highly Intelligent and Gifted Children); Zihinsel Yetersiz Çocukları

Family and Social Research (*T.C. Başbakanlık Aile ve Sosyal Araştırmalar Genel Müdürlüğü*) periodically conducts and publishes results on social research on the family and children. These include topics like child education in the family (1991), childcare problems of working mothers (1992), domestic violence (1997) and family structure and problems of Turks living in Germany (2005).

A number of studies have looked into the effects of media on children. Duran (2008) has examined how television news in general ignores the effect it has on children and comments on media ethics from the children's point of view; Tanrıöver (2008) has analysed how the popular TV film "*Kurtlar Vadisi*" influences 15–18-year-old boys and encourages more violent forms of resistance. Erjem (2008) has looked at the way daily newspapers focus on street children in their news, reinforcing the association between these children and crime; Kar (2008) has noted that Turkey is among the top three countries in television watching, and she has explored the influence TV channels have on socializing children to become avid consumers. Gürsoy (2009) has looked at Internet games, and reached the interesting conclusion that modern games, by allowing children to pick up different colours, enable them to select different paths through space. Comparable to the traditional Turkish games *Çömçe Bride*, they can have similarly constructive influences on child development. Onur (2005), writing about the psychosexual history of childhood and youth in Turkey, has compiled a collection of memoirs and writings exploring childhood experiences of sexuality and falling in love.

From a scholarly point of view, it may not be wrong to say that there are groundbreaking research studies focusing on children and childhood. Numerous research papers, reports, scientific articles, archive studies and ethnographies can be found relating to issues of childhood. These include the disciplines of anthropology, sociology, social work, criminology, psychology, psychiatry, law, folklore, literature and public health.

Numerous popular self-help books and studies dwell on childhood in Turkey. The psychiatrist Yörükoğlu and the psychologist Cüceloğlu have written prolifically about child psychology and the changes from a traditional patriarchal family to more nuclear-family-oriented lifestyles. From a humanitarian point of view, they dwell on the meaning of these changes. Authors like Tuzcuoğlu and Tuzcuoğlu (2004) focus on the sexual education of children. Writers like Mehmedoğlu (2005) combine knowledge of child psychology and apply this for the use of Islamic training and socialization.

Here I would like to cite in greater detail four examples of social research on childhood-related issues in the Turkish context. All four are critical of existing theories and argue for the need to introduce new scientific paradigms. The first two of these belong to Kağıtçıbaşı's works on child socialization and development. As the third, I would like to bring to attention Gürsoy's work on infant and child mortality in urban Istanbul. Fourth, I feel Delaney's ethnographic accounts of rural childhood

---

Yetiştirme ve Koruma Vakfı (ziçev) (Foundation for the Education and Protection of Mentally Inadequate Children).

experiences are revealing for understanding gender, religion and symbolic realms. I have given detailed accounts of Delaney's descriptions and analyses, because even though considerable attention is given to studies on Islam (see Religion Monitor, 2008), there are few studies on detailed childhood experiences of religion and how this influences life cognitively.

6 Kağıtçıbaşı's Model of Child Development and Personality Formation

As a social psychologist, Kağıtçıbaşı has been the first to write internationally on the influence of social change and westernization on child development and personality formation in Turkey. She has argued that with the trends towards individualism, the positive aspects of traditional modes of connectivity are being lost in the modern Turkish family. However, Kağıtçıbaşı (1996b) argues that there is an alternative path of development that would combine the best of two worlds:

> Autonomy is often construed as separateness from others and is seen to result from a separation-individuation process. However, it is neither logically nor psychologically necessary for autonomy to imply separateness if the existence of the two different dimensions of agency and interpersonal distance are recognized. The two poles of the agency dimension are autonomy and heteronomy; those of the interpersonal distance dimension are separateness and relatedness. The two dimensions are confused when agency is pitted against relatedness (p. 180).

Kağıtçıbaşı examines different family interaction models in terms of child-rearing patterns and the resultant types of (developing) selves. She suggests one of these, the autonomous-relational self, as a healthy synthesis of the two basic human needs for agency and relatedness. She argues that this tends to develop in the family model of emotional interdependence involving authoritative parenting. This family model and self-constellation, which is supported by research evidence, involve a different set of theories from those traditionally found in psychology. The conceptualization synthesizes some apparently conflicting patterns of interpersonal relations and the self. Kağıtçıbaşı believes this may serve as a corrective to the pervasive emphasis in psychology on individual autonomy at the cost of human relatedness (1996, p. 180).

Kağıtçıbaşı's other significant contribution to the field of childhood studies is the "Turkish Early Enrichment Project" (TEEP), which has been assessed by a follow-up study after 22 years. Kağıtçıbaşı et al. (2009) state that long-term studies of early intervention, spanning over decades, are scarce in the United States and nonexistent in the rest of the world, and that the TEEP is the only non-U.S. example to date. In a paper, they report a new follow-up assessment of the long-term outcomes of TEEP, an intervention carried out in 1983–1985 with 4–6-year-old children from deprived backgrounds. Previous evaluations had been carried out at the completion of the intervention and 7 years later. The findings from 131 of the original

255 participants indicated that children who received either mother training, educational preschool or both had more favourable outcomes in terms of educational attainment, occupational status, age of beginning gainful employment, and some indicators of integration into modern urban life such as owning a computer compared to those who had neither training. Further analyses of the intervention effects on the complete post-intervention developmental trajectories indicated that children whose cognitive deficits prior to the intervention were mild to moderate but not severe benefited from early enrichment. Thus, a majority of the children who received early enrichment had more favourable trajectories of development into young adulthood in the cognitive/achievement and social developmental domains than comparable children who did not receive enrichment (Kağıtçıbaşı et al., 2009).

7 Research on Infant and Child Mortality in Göçkent, Istanbul

Fortunately, child mortality has become a less prevalent public health problem in Turkey, but nevertheless, like the tip of an iceberg, it is still an important indicator of a multitude of social, cultural and environmental factors. The Göçkent research is significant from several points of view. As an anthropological study that has also used numerical data, the work demonstrates how qualitative and quantitative methods can complement each other and serve to illuminate paths of understanding that would not be possible with the use of only one methodological approach. Research on the cultural factors related to infant and child mortality, carried out in a low-income area of Istanbul (1986–1989), found that the most significant variables associated with child mortality were not attributes of the mother, but attributes of the father and characteristics of the household. After analysis of more than 500 variables for each woman interviewed, a multiple regression analysis revealed four variables that made the most significant contribution to explaining child mortality. These were, in order of significance, the father's education, the household composition, the mother's attitude towards abortion, and the amount of drinking and smoking by members of the family other than the mother. In view of these results, Gürsoy argued for the need to review the theoretical paradigm that necessitates an almost exclusive linkage of child health to a focus on mother-child bonding (Gürsoy, 1992a).

The Istanbul sample suggested two extreme types representing two different social environments in which children grow up. In the "bad cases", there is extreme patriarchal control of the woman in that she lives with her in-laws; her husband has poor education, and thus his dependency on his family is greater; she has internalized reproductive values that leave her little capacity for autonomy; and there is heavy drinking and smoking in the household. In contrast to this, in the "good cases", there is high education for fathers and, together with this, a separate, nuclear family residence into which babies are born. The woman's views on abortion are more liberal than religious or secular dictates, indicating a woman ready to try alternatives; and the household is free of the ill-effects of alcohol or cigarette consumption (Gürsoy, 1994, pp. 183–184). Thus, this research also argued for the need to free health issues from a strictly public health paradigm towards more creative, in-depth approaches in the use of introducing new, culturally appropriate concepts to discuss child health issues.

8 Rural Childhoods in Delaney's Ethnography

Based on participant observation in the early 1980s in rural Turkey, Delaney has written about semantic and other symbols used culturally in the socialization of Turkish children. Her observations reflect the meaning of childhood with its gender complexities embedded in cosmology. She notes that the word *çocuk* means both child and boy. When asked how many children they have, people in the village generally gave the number of boys. Girls in some important sense do not count; they are concealed linguistically just as their bodies are concealed beneath their baggy clothes, behind their veils, and within the house. *Çocuk* functions like the English "man"; it is both generic and gender-specific, and is often very difficult to determine which meaning is implied, a problem that confounds those who deal with historical or census documents (Delaney, 1991, p. 75).

Although the production of a child is synonymous with marriage, child is synonymous with son; therefore, women must continue to reproduce children until a son is born. Delaney (1991) takes a critical view of social studies on the value of children, and the relative value of sons and daughters:

> The focus in the cross-cultural study on the consciously expressed value of sons, whether in the form of providing labor and social security or raising woman's status in her husband's home, is myopic. Not only does it miss the forest for the trees, but it ignores the invisible but all-important root of the matter, the importance of seed. Since it is only men who are thought capable of transmitting the inextinguishable life in seed, it is necessary to produce a son in order that the line continue (p. 76).

Although a son is absolutely necessary to continue the family, children in general are a source of delight and the family's primary amusement. Children are considered a necessity for a happy life. They are both distracting and a distraction; life without a child is considered dull and tasteless. Although everyone would like to have more land, more goods, and so on, such things are not considered as essential in the way that children are. They are essential not only for a complete life, but also to complete the socialization of their parents. A person without a child has not fulfilled the purpose for which he or she was created, and thus is still unfinished. Such a person is considered neither responsible nor fully adult (Delaney, 1991, p. 76).

Delaney's observations lead her to conclude that babies are viewed as the most immature persons. They are like toys; they are picked up, fondled, and transferred from person to person throughout the day (Delaney, 1991, p. 77). She observes that children are said to not possess reason and therefore cannot be reasoned with. Adults rarely tried to offer children rational arguments for or against certain behaviours. Undesirable behaviours were called *ayıp* (shameful), but the child was not really held responsible; in fact, what is undesirable seemed to depend not on the actions themselves but on the context. Sometimes and in some places, certain actions were more annoying than in others. Discipline was relatively arbitrary, as were rewards. When children did something that annoyed their parents, they were yelled at or given a light slap but were rarely beaten.

Delaney notes that children were indulged and spoiled. They were given anything they saw and asked for, not just in order to pacify them but because it was believed to be sinful and greedy to withhold something from a child. Children cannot be held responsible for making unreasonable demands; things they should not have ought to be hidden, "covered". Thus people delivering food or other items to a neighbour covered them so that all the children in the street would not ask for a share. She observes that girls were spoiled even more than boys, not because they were seen as more valuable than boys, but precisely because they were seen as less valuable. Girls are merely guests for a brief time in their parents' home; they are *el* (foreign, outsiders), as they will also be in their husband's house. She concludes that as children, boys are much more constrained by the notions of respect and deference to elders; at the same time, this demeanour is an expression of their own worth (Delaney, 1991, p. 78).

9 Childhood Is Sinless: Childhood Paralleled in Cosmology

Delaney continues to note that although the present schedule of the *ezan* (Muslim call to prayer) does punctuate the work day, perhaps it is also a recognition that the times of the day are not uniform: that a day, like a life, has its own rhythms. Perhaps it is an icon marking life's stages. The long morning period may represent the blank, sinless period of childhood until marriage, the noontime of life, after which it becomes more important to consider the things of the spirit, for one becomes accountable, and sins are more likely to accumulate. The last two *ezan*, close together in the evening, may be a reminder that at the end of life, before one enters the long sleep, one's mind ought to be even more turned to God. The notion of "turning" is important in Turkish Islam, and is given physical expression in the movements of the Mevlana or Whirling Dervishes.

Delaney picks up an interesting cultural detail when she notes that in the village, the scene of Abraham's intended sacrifice is visually prominent, being displayed on posters, wall hangings and post cards. In all these representations, a boy is tied hand and foot like a sheep, while his father stands over him brandishing a knife in an upraised hand. She wonders how this is internalized; what kinds of sentiments are generated in children. Delaney (1991, p. 300) asks whether witnessing the sacrifice helps to strengthen and reinforce authoritarian values.[4]

---

[4]She further notes that in the Old Testament, Abraham assumed the right to dispose of his son without consulting his wife, Sarah, or asking for her consent. Nor did God speak to her. Clearly, the child was not hers in the same sense; in other words, once again the theory of procreation is crucial to understanding the story. Philosophical commentaries on this story talk about the child as Abraham's dearest possession. Clearly, if the child was a possession, Abraham did not need permission to dispose of him as he wished; he had the *patria potestas*, the power, and the right of the father (Delaney, 1991, p. 301).

10 Urban Childhoods in Memoirs, Diaries and Autobiographies

Novels, memoirs and diaries give us refined accounts of the world of children. To my knowledge, there are no published diaries written by children in Turkey. However, many writers have given us rich descriptions of their experiences and data on childhood in the form of novels, autobiographies and memoirs.[5] These accounts give details of children's play, relationships with family and friends, memoirs of loss of family members, remarriage of parents, religious rituals and practices, migration, war, poverty and milestone experiences shaping one's identity.

Karaca Taşkent, who funded and published the popular *Doğan Kardeş* (Brother Doğan) children's magazine (1945–1974) in Turkey, has written about his elder brother Doğan who died in an avalanche in the Alps in Switzerland in 1939, while attending a boarding school:

> Ever since I remember myself, I knew of the death of my elder brother. But I do not recollect his death, or those days. Very vaguely I can remember a picture. In the old wooden house, in the middle room, we had cubes with pictures on them. When you turn around the cubes the pictures change... We were playing with those cubes. He has remained in my imagination like such a vision. I do not remember anything else (Söğüt, 2003, p. 23).

In her memoirs, the famous Turkish sociologist Abadan-Unat (2003), born in Vienna in 1921 as the daughter of an aristocratic Austrian mother and an Ottoman father, writes that she is trying to force her memory to reach out to her first recollections, to try to remember the first environment, the people that shaped the first imprints of her identity:

> I must have come to the age of six. With my white fur hat and coat, I was taken to a photographer. According to what my aunt says, one day my father took this photograph to my grandmother... and said, "And what do you say to this?" My grandmother, who despite having spent all her adult life in İzmir, could never forget Bosnia Herzegovina where she was born and raised, took a look at the picture and said (in Bosnian) "My son, what concern is this infidel bastard kid to me?" A great silence fell into the room. Five minutes later, my father composed himself and could say, "But she is your grand child". After another long five minutes the response came, "Then bring them to Turkey" (pp. 15–21).

In his memoirs, Pamuk (2003) recounts his early childhood experiences of sexuality, his fantasies of imaginary friends and his feelings of secret and puzzling relations with other people, and comments, "The difference between the man who constantly thinks that he is Napoleon and the man who fantasizes that he is Napoleon is the difference between the unhappy schizophrenic and the happy fantasizer" (p. 28).

As Fernea (2002) points out, childhood memoirs are private recollections and adult constructions of childhood experience and existence. They give us a personal understanding of who the adult writers are and what they have become, seen through the prism of childhoods remembered. They are excursions into personal

---

[5]To name a few among many, see Ağaoğlu (2004), Göze (2007), Güvenç (2004), Tarzi (1993), Taşkent cited in Söğüt (2003).

pasts, journeys to childhood homelands. Differences and complexities of gender, class, ethnicity, nationality and religious background shape the nature of experiences. This paradox gains additional dimension when we move out of our own cultural environment and into the less familiar territory of other cultural settings.

Furthermore, childhood memoirs written by adults are not children speaking as children but adults reconstructing their childhood remembrances through the prism of time. Often the recollections of childhood are based on accounts of what older relatives and acquaintances have told, in many cases repeatedly, and what is later remembered selectively. As with any autobiography, the reality of having authors speaking about themselves gives a special authority to what they say, but at the same time, the narratives and personal histories are selected, constructed and targeted for the consumption of a particular audience. Therefore, such autobiographical writings need to be viewed critically before being taken to be the "voices of children" (Fernea, 2002, pp. 1–5).

11 Prejudices, Discrimination, Present Day Islamophobia and Beyond

Finally, I would like to comment on discrimination and prejudices in the context of Turkish children. The report of the World Federation for Mental Health (WFMH) in the follow-up and implementation of the "Durban Declaration on Racism, Racial Discrimination, Xenophobia and Related Forms of Intolerance" states that in recent years, reported acts of incitement to racial, ethnic and religious hatred have increased dramatically in the world, and that in all continents, vulnerable communities—especially members of minorities—are victims of public utterances calling for intolerance and discrimination and, in some cases, physical and psychological violence.

The report recognizes the lack of recognition of multiculturalism as an underlying factor of racism and the central issue in present-day crises in most regions of the world. The report states that although societies are the outcome of lengthy historical processes involving contact between peoples, cultures and religions, the central problem of most modern societies lies in the fundamental contradiction between the framework of the nation state, the expression of an exclusive national identity and the dynamics of multiculturalization. Even the concept of multiculturalism, the predominant model for the integration of foreigners or minorities, is criticized on the grounds that it serves as a fantasy screen for the indigenous or dominant group to sustain their libidinal economies around a notion of alterity. The terms are used in a dialectical fashion to conceal their continued hold on power in relations to immigrant minorities (Lanz, 2009, pp. 7–8).

Furthermore, as Hall (2005) points out, social learning theories suggest that attitudes such as prejudice are learned in childhood through contact with older and influential figures who reward children (with, for example, love and praise) for adopting their views. It is suggested that children as young as 3 years of age are aware of two of the major social categories, namely gender and ethnicity, and from that age on, can readily identify with some categories rather than others and demonstrate clear attitudinal and behavioural preferences. Studies show that children also adapt and conform to the social norms of the group to which they belong, resulting in the development and expression of prejudicial attitudes towards others (Hall, 2005, p. 31).

How are Turkish children affected by prejudices, racism and xenophobia? We need to pose several questions: First, how are Turkish children living in Europe affected by prejudice and discrimination against them?[6] How is the Islamophobia since 9/11 affecting the lives of Muslim children the world over (Kaya, 2009, p. 383)? The autobiography of the former gang member Cem Gülay and the foreword written by his cousin, who is presently a member of the Berlin City Parliament, reveal how discrimination by teachers and classmates in schools can lead to rebellion and anti-social and criminal behaviour in children and youth (Hürriyet, 2009). In a questionnaire administered to representatives of Turkish NGOs in Holland, the worst problem they expressed was failure at school (38.9%), and thus related to children. This was only followed in second place by unemployment (24.1%) (see Küçükcan/Veyis, 2009, p. 53). The literature shows that Turkish immigrants in the European Union have had to face many forms of discrimination and hostility. The situation appears to have worsened whenever there were perceptions of economic crisis, particularly in the 1980s, 1990s and presently as a result of Islamophobia. A rise in the number of violent attacks on foreigners, particularly on Turks, has a detrimental effect on what are already victimized communities. Although various laws prohibiting violence and overt discrimination on racial grounds exist in many European countries, it is accepted that practices and attitudes, which may have the same effect, often persist in subtler and disguised forms (Çiçekçi 1998, p. 49). These may have particularly negative effects for girls, particularly those wearing head scarves, because they become symbols of "the other" (see Koç, 2009, p. 119).

We may also distinguish other forms of discrimination, albeit in scientific discourse and terminology. For example, in a workshop report funded by the European Science Foundation entitled "Changing Childhood in a Changing Europe", the authors make it look like the real situation of insufficient research on children of Turkish origin is actually a situation in which they take an unfair portion of the cake: "In studies on migration and integration in general, it is often the respective major immigrant groups which get more or less all the attention—like Turks and repatriates of German origin in the case of Germany" (Knörr, 2009, p. 27).

Yet another question arises when issues of children of low-income groups or minorities are conceptualized and discussed without the inclusion of children of dominant or high-income groups. For example, researchers in the Department of Social Medicine at Harvard Medical School published a text report, called "World Mental Health". The sub-title of the book is "Problems and Priorities in Low-Income Countries" (Desjarlais, Eisenberg, Good, & Kleinman, 1995). The work has a

---

[6]There are about 3.6 million Turkish citizens living throughout the world in more than 30 countries including Saudi Arabia, the USA, Australia, the Russian Federation, Kuwait and Japan (Harding, 2007, pp. 485–486).

separate chapter on "Children and Youth". Even though the study recognizes that nearly all mental health problems addressed in the report occur in both low-income and high-income societies, the authors nevertheless, by separating the analysis of culture-specifically appropriate prevention programmes and policies, fail to see the interconnectedness of and the influence of international relations and conflict in child mental health issues.

In addition to popular or scientifically constructed discrimination against Turkish children, we also need to address the question of discriminatory patterns within Turkish society itself. In addition to issues of class, gender, age and ethnicity, social scientists also need to recognize and address forms of discrimination that develop towards communities with different modes of livelihood. Turkey has a small population of *Yörük* nomads, their numbers estimated to be only in thousands. Similar to many other nation states with nomadic populations, the state in Turkey has tried to get these communities to settle down and become agriculturalists. Nomadic populations often have more adverse public health problems; the schooling of children is problematic; it is difficult to hold a registry of the population and more difficult to monitor the population for security reasons. Such groups are viewed with suspicion by the settled villagers as well as town people. What issues do nomadic children face? Nomadic youth and adults say that they would rather enjoy the freedom of open landscapes, spaces and movement. They find cities interesting, attractive but undesirable for living in. Do nomadic children have to leave their lifestyle behind in order to find social acceptance, better health and education?

Recently, a study was conducted by the Jewish community of Turkey to assess the image of Jews in Turkey. What does it mean to be a child of a less dominant group within Turkey or among Turks? The research showed that even when people have never met a member of one group, there can nevertheless be fears and a desire for distance (*Radikal*, 3 October 2009).

To present the complexity of conflicts and trends impacting on children and child socialization, I would like to add the fear of globalization and the reaction to westernization that some groups perceive to be a post-modern form of destructive colonization. This process is seen to be more sinister than colonization by physical force and military measures. The target is the minds and brains of the young children, who instead of learning their traditional and national legends and stories like *Keloğlan, Nasreddin Hodja, Köroğlu, Aşık Kerem* and *Karacaoğlan* start to become familiar with Mickey Mouse, the Flintstones, Jay R, Lord of the Rings and Harry Potter. Traditional cultural values are thus replaced by the dominance of other values. Instead of collective values saying "one of us for all of us; all of us for one of us", the new values dictate, "down with the downtrodden". Babies grow up with English lullabies, and thus their national genetic code is altered (Özbek, 2007, p. 52).

12 Conclusion

It is not possible to give a final word on all the issues raised in this paper. More than anything, the objective has been to highlight relevant questions. Childhood studies in Turkey have a prolific background embedded in the traditional and historical value attributed to children. There are more than 70 Turkish proverbs and sayings related to children and childhood (Albayrak, 2009, pp. 306–309). It can be said that Sunay Akın's toy museum in Istanbul (*Istanbul Oyuncak Müzesi*) is a living example of the attention devoted to childhood in present-day Turkey. An internationally comparative evaluation of norms, values and theories developed to assess the world of children, coupled with new developments in our understanding of childhood, would add further dimensions to social studies focusing on children in Turkey. Given the space allocated to children in many different scientific disciplines, one can argue for the establishment of academic programmes on childhood in the country. Such an interdisciplinary focus on childhood could lead to master's or PhD degrees, and such academic research, strengthened by international collaboration, could, in turn, help to illuminate our relationship with children and with the different life stages of humanity throughout the world.

References

Abadan-Unat, N. (2003). *Kum Saatini İzlerken* (Memoirs). Istanbul: İletişim.

Ağaoğlu, S. (2004). *Bir Ömür Böyle Geçti* (Memoirs). Istanbul: İshak Basımevi.

Albayrak, N. (2009). Türkiye Türkcesinden Atasözleri. Istanbul: Kapı Yayınları.

Ariés, P. (1962). *Centuries of childhood*. London: Penguin Books.

Çiçekli, B. (1998). *The legal position of Turkish immigrants in the European Union*. Ankara: Karmap.

Delaney, C. (1991). *The seed and the soil: Gender & cosmology in Turkish village society*. Berkeley, CA: University of California Press.

Desjarlais, R., Eisenberg, L., Good, B., & Kleinman, A. (1995). *World mental health – Problems and priorities in low-income countries*. Oxford: Oxford University Press.

Duran, R. (2008). Çocuk ve Medya. In G. İnceoğlu & N. Akıner (Eds.), *Medya ve Çocuk Rehberi*. Konya: Eğitim Kitabevi.

Erjem, Y. (2008). Medya ve Sokak Çocukları. In G. İnceoğlu & N. Akıner (Eds.), *Medya ve Çocuk Rehberi*. Konya: Eğitim Kitabevi.

European Science Foundation, Setting Science Agendas for Europe. (2009). *Changing childhood in a changing Europe*. Interdisciplinary Workshop Report.

Fernea, E. W. (Ed.). (2002). *Remembering childhood in the Middle East: Memoirs from a century of change*. Austin, TX: University of Texas Press.

Göze, H. (2007). *Kadıköylü Yıllarım, Çocukluk ve Gençlik Hatıralarım*. Istanbul: Kubbealtı Yayınları.

Gürsoy, A. (1992a). Infant mortality: A Turkish puzzle? *Health Transition Review, 2*(2), 131–149.

Gürsoy, A. (1992b) Introduction. In A. Ören (Ed.), *Please, no police. Series of Middle Eastern fiction in translation*. Austin, TX: University of Texas Press.

Gürsoy, A. (1994). Forum: Parental education and child mortality. *Health Transition Review, 4*(2), 183–185.

Gürsoy, A. (1995a). The changing discourse on childhood in Turkey. In E. W. Fernea (Ed.), *Children in the Muslim Middle East*. Austin, TX: University of Texas Press.

Gürsoy, A. (1995b). Traditional practices affecting the health of women and children. In O. Neyzi (Ed.), *The basics of maternal and child health*. Ankara: Çocuk Sağlığı Enstitüsü-UNICEF.

Gürsoy, A. (1996a). Abortion in Turkey: A matter of state, family or individual decision. *Social Science and Medicine, 42*(4), 531–542.

Gürsoy, A. (1996b). Beyond the orthodox: Heresy in medicine and the social sciences from a cross-cultural perspective. *Social Science and Medicine, 43*(5), 577–599.

Gürsoy, A. (1996c). Letter to the editor. *Social Science and Medicine, 42*(4), 479–482.

Gürsoy, A. (1998). Sections 4, 7 and 16 on health, youth, & beauty; migration; planning the population. In *Üç Kuşak Cumhuriyet*. Istanbul: Turkish Economic and Social History Foundation.

Gürsoy, A. B. (2009). Çömçe Gelinden Dijital Oyunlara. In A. B. Gürsoy (Ed.), *Medya İncelemeleri*. Istanbul: Es Yayınları.

Güvenç, B. (2004). *Anılardan Sayfalar*. Istanbul: İş Bankası Kültür Yayınları.

Hacettepe University Institute of Population Studies. (2009). *Türkiye – Nüfus ve Sağlık Araştırması*. Ankara, Turkey.

Hall, N. (2005). *Hate crime*. Cullompton: Willan Publishing.

Harding, Ç. (2007). Yurtdışındaki Çağdaş Türk Toplumları. In D. Kuban (Ed.), *Türkçe Konuşanlar* (pp. 485–495). Tetragon: Prince Claus Fund Library.

Hürriyet. (2009, October 26). *Daily Turkish Newspaper*. Istanbul, Turkey.

Kağıtçıbaşı, Ç. (1996a). *Family and human development across cultures: A view from the other side*. Hillsdale, NJ: Erlbaum.

Kağıtçıbaşı, Ç. (1996b). The autonomous-relational self: A new synthesis. *European Psychologist, 1*(3), 180–186.

Kağıtçıbaşı, Ç., Sunar, D., Bekman, S., Baydar, N., & Camalcılar, Z. (2009). Continuing effects of early enrichment in adult life: The Turkish Early Enrichment Project 22 years later. *Journal of Applied Developmental Psychology*. doi: 10.1016/j.appdev.2009.05.03

Kar, A. (2008). Çocuk Tüketiciler ve Tüketilen Çocukluk. In G. İnceoğlu & N. Akıner (Eds.), *Medya ve Çocuk Rehberi*. Konya: Eğitim Kitabevi.

Kaya, P. (2009). Euro-Turks and the European Union: Migration, Islam and the reign of fear. In T. Küçükcan & G. Veyis (Eds.), *Turks in Europe – Culture, identity, integration* (pp. 383–410). Amsterdam: Turkevi Research Centre.

Koç, G. (2009). Turks in Austria and Germany: Stereotypes and xenophobia. In T. Küçükcan & G. Veyis (Eds.), *Turks in Europe – Culture, identity, integration* (pp. 103–127). Amsterdam: Turkevi Research Centre.

Küçükcan, T. & Veyis, G. (Eds.)(2009). *Turks in Europe – Culture, identity, integration* (pp. 383–410). Amsterdam: Turkevi Research Centre.

Lanz, T. (2009). Turkish immigrants in Germany: Behind the fantasy screen of multiculturalism. In T. Küçükcan & G. Veyis (Eds.), *Turks in Europe – Culture, identity, integration* (pp. 7–34). Amsterdam: Turkevi Research Centre.

Mead, M. (1970). Our educational emphases in primitive perspective. In J. Middleton (Ed.), *From child to adult*. Austin, TX: University of Texas Press. (Original work published in 1941).

Mehmedoğlu, Y. (2005). Ahlaki ve Dini Gelişim. Çocuğum Değerlerimizi Öğreniyor. Morpa Kültür Yayinlari

Onur, B. (2005). *Anılardaki Aşklar, Çocukluğun ve Gençliğin Psikoseksüel Tarihi*. Istanbul: KitapYayınevi.

Özbek, H. (2007). *İngilizce Ninnilerle Uyutayım Seni, Büyüteyim Seni, Eğiteyim Seni*. Istanbul: Kumsaati Yayınları.

Pamuk, O. (2003). *Istanbul – Hatıralar ve Şehir*. Istanbul: İletişim.

Perrig-Chiello (2009). European Child Cohort Network (EUCCONET). An ESF Research Networking Programme. *Changing Childhood in a Changing Europe*. Strasbourg.

Reddy, N. M. (1988). Twenty stories by Turkish women writers. *Indiana University Turkish Studies*, 8.

Şehsuvaroğlu, B. (1984). *Türk Tıp Tarihi*. Bursa: Taş.

Söğüt, M. (2003). *Sevgili Doğan Kardeş*. Turkey: Yapı Kredi Yayınları.

Tanrıöver, H. (2008). „Vadi"de Büyüyen Erkek Çocuklar. In G. İnceoğlu & N. Akıner (Eds.), *Medya ve Çocuk Rehberi*. Konya: Eğitim Kitabevi.

Tarzi, P. (1993). *Anılar*. Istanbul: Omaş Ofset.

Turkish Bureau of Statistics (TÜİK). Data taken from address-based census records (ADNKS) 2008, http://tuik.gov.tr/reports

Tuzcuoğlu, N & Tuzcuoğlu, S. (2004). Çocuğun Cinsel Eğitimi – Anne, Ben Nasıl Doğdum?. İstanbul: Morpa Kültür Yayınları, 2. Baskı.

Part IV
Structural Conditions and Children in Different National Contexts

Tim Köhler and Uwe Sander

1 Introduction

International childhood and child studies from a so-called western perspective are confronted with the problem of making comparisons between criteria that are assumed to represent objective conditions for all the children to be surveyed. This raises the concern that they take a culturalist approach, especially when studying the children's conception of well-being and a good life. The central aims when analysing children's well-being are to gain information on their subjective preferences and opinions. However, these cannot be separated from their life conditions that differ significantly both within and between nation states. Although every child has to deal with individual conditions, their broader environment embedded in the political system represented by the nation state also plays an important role. Despite the decline or liberalisation of the welfare state (Esping-Andersen, 1997), the political process and possible actions are still concentrated on the level of this system in which political changes have to be initiated to accomplish better conditions for a good life or to ensure the existence of positive structures.

Currently, the international debate can be seen as a host of different national approaches that contribute to diverse criteria for childhood and child studies. The following section presents a blend of different national approaches to children's well-being and points out relevant categories. The chapters present methodological and systematic approaches that may be of benefit for the construction of an international study designed to analyse children's attitude towards a good life.

Research taking an international perspective has to tackle not only political, social or economic differences but also theoretical problems. This is why most of the relevant studies concentrate on a limited investigation area (e.g. Brandolini and D'Alessio, 1998) or on limited indicators and methodological issues associated with "child well-being" (Brown, 2008). As a result, they present a collection of different

T. Köhler (✉)
Faculty of Educational Science, Bielefeld University, 33615 Bielefeld, Germany
e-mail: tim.koehler3@uni-bielefeld.de

dimensions, but not a "complete picture". Childhood and child studies like the World Vision study (Andresen and Hurrelmann, 2007) cover different perspectives, but are unable to integrate the whole theme. Even the definitions and factors of well-being are controversial, and the operationalisations for studying children's individual conceptions of well-being are wide ranging (Ben-Arieh, 2005). In addition, childhood and social theory are essentially controversial fields (Alanen, 1997; Honig, 1999; Nussbaum, 2000; Rawls, 1975; Sen, 1999).

One possible link between these dimensions could be a conjunctive approach such as the Capabilities Approach (Albus et al., 2009, see also the article by Holger Ziegler in this volume). Every integrative approach and also any operationalisation in an international child study has to tackle the problem of rebinding existing theories and methods that may well differ in their current national approaches and contexts. These contexts create the challenges confronting any ambitious international project on children's individual conceptions of a good life.

The following section deals with some of the main global conditions resulting from recent social and economic processes. Although the different nation states have different starting conditions, effects are similar: an increasing problem of poverty and inequality among children. In addition, internal and extraterritorial migration have not declined during the course of globalisation, and ethnicity continues to be a central theme.

Migration and its potential for conflict and as a subject of inequality can be identified as one of the central issues in the national problematisation of childhood. It uncovers the underlying problems of social inequality and poverty and their outcome for growing-up in a significant way, and it used to be one of the main indicators for international research. This is reflected in the different problematisations applied by all the following authors. The transformation problems show the outcome of centuries of migration and the still important role of ethnicity, especially in the former Soviet Union and eastern parts of Europe. One perspective deals with the transformation of the state, including social conflicts generated by inequality and problems of inclusion for the whole population and the way these influence children's possible chances for a good life. The increasing gap between the rich and poor is hardly balanced by social rights (Marshall, 1950), and underlying conflicts of ethnic, regional or social origins emerge. The global phenomenon of migration corresponded with the political and social changes until the late 1980s. This is expressed in the following articles that deal with the central connection between market strategies, the decline of the welfare state and the changing conditions of childhood and youth.

In addition to these more or less political problems, another relevant criterion is the demographic differences in the analysed states. In Turkey, for example, the percentage of children is much higher than in other countries such as Germany. Age structure is one of the dominant differences between the populations of the countries. As a result the demographic categories and their social and political outcomes are outlined as main categories for an international study.

The political, social and scientific connection between poverty and the well-being of children can be found in different national perspectives. Although there are differences in national semantics, problems and levels of children's appraisal of the good life, one can see structural convergences referring to socioeconomic status. Despite changing values, the different national semantics show that there is an ubiquitary problem across other differentiation categories. The multidimensional pauperisation or a lack of social resources is to be seen in all countries, despite the variety of state interventions in their social systems.

This research reveals that the problem is primarily one of action and a lack of political will to change the situation, especially for risk groups. This problem is aggravated in terms of another relevant indicator for the well-being of children: their health. This highlights the two dimensions of individual and social categories. It also shows the need for research on children's attitudes towards a good life to combine qualitative and quantitative perspectives in order to identify structures and individual purposes. The individual characteristic of differentiated capitals (Bourdieu, 1979) is a perspective pointing towards the connections between the children's social and material environment and their subjective attitude towards a good life (Nussbaum, 2000; Sen, 1999), and it shows the necessity for combined analyses based on subjective and intersubjective methods.

The output of research on children's well-being and good life should also lead to concrete policy demands. The section shows that child poverty, migration, health and so forth are not only symbols of inequality and indicators of good life conditions (Clark and McGillivray, 2007), but also concrete dimensions for the individual chances and possibilities of achieving one's own conception of well-being. In future research, the different national semantics and approaches will have to deal with related criteria and problems that are relevant conditions for the realisation of well-being. To combine the different approaches and existing results will be one of the main tasks in light of the increasing global character of national challenges. Every process and social condition embraced in research must be examined within the context of globalisation and its social and political implications.

References

Alanen, L. (1997). Soziologie der Kindheit als Projekt: Perspektiven für die Forschung. *Zeitschrift für Sozialisationsforschung und Erziehungssoziologie, 17*(2), 162–177.

Albus, S., Andresen, S., Fegter, S., & Richter, M. (2009). Wohlergehen und das "gute Leben" in der Perspektive von Kindern. Das Potenzial des Capability Approach für die Kindheitsforschung. *Themenschwerpunkt der Zeitschrift für Soziologie der Erziehung und Sozialisation, 28*(3), 346–358.

Andresen, S., & Hurrelmann, K. (2007). *Kinder in Deutschland 2007. 1. World Vision Kinderstudie.* Frankfurt am Main: Fischer.

Ben-Arieh, A. (2005). Where are the children? Children's role in measuring and monitoring their well-being. *Social Indicators Research, 74*(3), 573–596.

Bourdieu, P. (1979). *La distinction. Critique sociale du jugement.* Paris: Minuit.

Brandolino, A., & D'Alessio, G. (1998). *Measuring well-being in the functioning space.* Rome: Mimeo, Branca d'Italia.

Brown, B. V. (Ed.). (2008). *Key indicators of child and youth well-being. Completing the picture,* New York: Taylor and Francis.

Clark, D., & McGillivray, M. (2007). Measuring human well-being: Key findings and policy lessons. (UNU Policy Brief No. 3). Helsinki, Finland. Accessed September 17, 2007, from http://www.wider.unu.edu/events/re search-presentations/book-launches/en_GB

Esping-Andersen, G. (1997). *The three worlds of welfare capitalism.* Cambridge: Polity Press.

Honig, M.-S. (1999). *Entwurf einer Theorie der Kindheit.* Frankfurt am Main: Suhrkamp.

Marshall, T. H. (1950). *Citizenship and social class.* Cambridge: Cambridge University Press.

Nussbaum, M. (2000). *Woman and human development. The capabilities approach.* Cambridge: Cambridge University Press.

Rawls, J. (1975). *Eine Theorie der Gerechtigkeit.* Frankfurt am Main: Suhrkamp.

Sen, A. (1999). *Development as freedom.* Oxford: Oxford University Press.

Child Poverty—Social and Economic Policy for Children

Antje Richter-Kornweitz

1 Spreading of Poverty

Although the unemployment rate in the European Union (EU) decreased in 2007 compared to 2005, families with unemployed persons and children have benefited little from this. The latest data shows that 16% of Europeans are still threatened by poverty, and the number of "working poor" also remains high (8% of workers are still poor, although they have a job).

In the EU-27, living in poverty is defined as earning less than 8,368 Euros a year as a person living alone (eurostat, Destatis, 2009). In Germany, the poverty line is a yearly income of less than 9,370 Euros. This puts Germany in 12th place among the EU states.

However, statistics vary. Depending on the basis of calculation, between 13% (European Union Statistics on Income and Living Conditions, 2006) and 18% (Sozio-oekonomisches Panel, 2006) of the total population in Germany were living in poverty in 2006. It is the children who are most affected. In the EU-27, children are more likely to live in poverty than the rest of the population (19%). According to the German SOEP (Socio-Economic Panel), the proportion of poor children up to 15 years of age in Germany was considerably higher than the EU average, with 26% in 2005 compared to 12% in the European Union Statistics on Income and Living Conditions (EU-SILC) in the same year. This figure rises steadily according to the SOEP (Schäfer, 2008). The OECD analysis (2008) confirms this tragedy for Germany, especially since 2000 and in comparison with other nations. Since then, the country in which inequality has most increased compared to all other OECD countries is Germany.

About one child in six (16.6%) or about 2 million children under 15 live on Hartz IV[1] in Germany (3. Armuts- und Reichtumsbericht der Bundesregierung, 2008).

A. Richter-Kornweitz (✉)
Federal State Association for Health and Academy for Social Medicine Lower Saxony (LVGAFS), 30165 Hannover, Germany
e-mail: antje.richter@gesundheit-nds.de

[1] Hartz IV is a financial subsistence benefit allocated by the government.

S. Andresen et al. (eds.), *Children and the Good Life*, Children's Well-Being: Indicators and Research 4, DOI 10.1007/978-90-481-9219-9_12,
© Springer Science+Business Media B.V. 2010

This does not include the children living in the families of the "working poor". Welfare organisations report that at least 2.5 million children in Germany live in poverty. In some regions, cities and parts of towns, every second or third child is poor. The children of single parents (38.2% with one child in the family), of unemployed parents (48%) or migrant parents (30%) are most affected. And more than 900,000 teenagers and young adults between 15 and 24 years themselves receiving Hartz IV in June 2008 add to this gloomy picture (Adamy, 2008).

2 Children with a Migration Background

In Germany around 6 million (27.2%) of the under-25-year-olds and 32.5% of the under-6-year-olds have a migration background—although more than 90% of them were born in Germany. According to the First World Vision Study, children with a migration background are much more likely to belong to socially deprived groups. Moreover, the number of parents with a migration background who subjectively consider their monthly income as insufficient is disproportionably high at 21% (Hurrelmann & Andresen, 2007).

Data from the Robert-Koch Institute's KiGGS study on youth health also offers specific evidence on the social status of girls and boys with a migration background. According to this study and its participants, youths with a double migration background are twice as likely to be in a socially deprived situation compared to those with no or only a single migration background (KiGG, 2008).

3 Life in Permanent Poverty

Marginalisation and a lack of equal opportunities are among the most important characteristics of poverty in German society. Children and teenagers growing up in poverty clearly have less access to established values, goods and to support services for youth. Their situation leads to undersupply in many fields.

When considering the age group of youth and the psychosocial effects of poverty on this group, one crucial aspect is whether this situation particularly affects the financial side, or whether the children and/or their families suffer from multidimensional and serious deprivation in several central areas of life. If several risks come together, such as teenage parenthood, illness of parents or divorce/separation, one can talk about a cumulation of poverty risks. This usually relates to a considerable burden on a child's development.

Permanently living under the poverty line creates a gap compared to the general living standard and imposes limitations on participation opportunities and equal participation. This also triggers considerable risks for the child's development opportunities. According to the European definition, people "permanently lacking income" are those who have less than 60% net equivalency income of the "medians", both currently and at least over the last two or three preceding years. A growing group of people in Europe are in this situation, but it is children who are especially strongly represented among them.

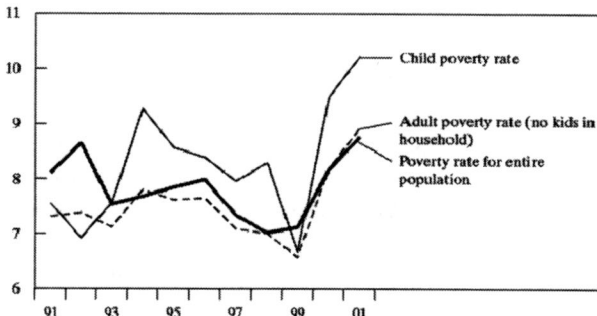

Fig. 1 Child versus other poverty rates (*Note*: Taken from Corak et al. for UNICEF 2005)

Corak, Fertig and Tamm (2005) drew on the SOEP to predict the future development of child poverty for UNICEF. It is remarkable how steeply child poverty rises compared to other population groups—another indicator that this phenomenon impacts particularly on children, that is to say, families with children (see Fig. 1).

Fertig and Tamm (2007, 2008) have also examined the dynamics of transition from poverty to non-poverty. They found that the length of time people remain poor is increasing, and that it particularly hits children of single parents. The situation has worsened just as much for children in immigrant families since the mid-1990s. Since then, they have been affected considerably more by poverty than children who have no migration background. The situation looks brighter for children of single parents who work full time and have higher qualifications. This combination of features influences the poverty experience more than the nationality.

4 Poverty as a Developmental Risk

Poverty has to be perceived as a risk to development. This applies to the degree of social integration as well as participation rates in central areas of life such as health and education. The social status of boys and girls determines whether they have access to these basic goods. Children with low social status are deprived, undersupplied and subject to strains in different areas that have a negative effect on mental/emotional and physical development, social integration, education and basic provisions, as Table 1 shows.

Table 1 Economic situation of the household (family poverty)

Dimensions of the basis of life of the child	
Material situation of child	Provision of basic supplies (e.g. shelter, nutrition, clothing)
"Provision" in the cultural field	Education (e.g. work, play and speech behaviour)
Social situation	Social integration (e.g. contacts, social skills)
Mental and physical situation	Health (e.g. health status, physical development)

Note: Taken from Hock and Holz (1999).

5 Child Poverty and Health

Social inequality impacts on the health status of the individual and leads to health inequality over the life course. Results of national and international studies, as well as continuous monitoring investigations, reveal a difference between health levels depending on social status. The studies name—ostentatiously said—the significant relationship between material poverty, education and health. They clearly prove that social inequality leads to health inequality through differences in health-related factors (e.g. gender), and thereby also to differences in morbidity and mortality. Empirical analyses over the whole life span confirm a lower life expectancy for men (of 10 years) and women (of 8 years) in the lowest compared to the highest status group (see Fig. 2).

The difference between health levels depending on social status starts to increase in early youth. The unequal health opportunities of socially deprived children are apparent at an early stage in the development of the senses of sight and hearing, oral health and several other areas. There is also an increased risk of early developmental disorders, deficits in physical exercise and eating behaviour, being overweight and smoking, as well as mental and behavioural differences (13. Kinder- und Jugendbericht 2009; Hurrelmann, Klocke, Melzer & Ravens-Sieberer, 2003; KiGGS, 2008; Mielk, 2000, 2004, 2008; Richter, Holz & Altgeld, 2004; Rosenbrock, 2004; Schlack, 2003).

The 11th youth report of the German government notes that the lower social layers are disproportionally affected not only by so-called learning disabilities but also by almost all types of disability (Beck, 2002). Summarising, it can be said that growing up in poverty increases how pronounced deficits and disorders are. Its consequences can be learning disability but also language disabilities and behavioural disorders and disabilities with organic, mental, physical or sense-specific causes (Weiß, 2000).

It is assumed that one reason for these outcomes is a lack of resources. A reason for delayed treatment may be parents who lack assertiveness when it comes to

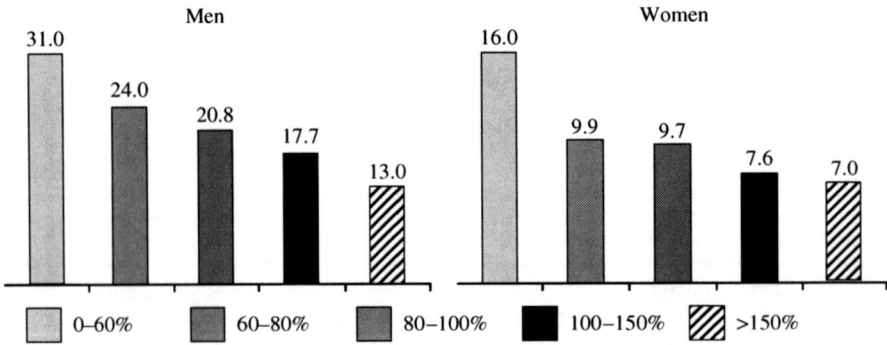

Fig. 2 Early mortality before age 65 by income and gender (*Note*: Data from SOEP and mortality tables for 1995–2005. Taken from Lampert, Kroll & Dunkelberg, 2007)

getting the necessary treatments or also lack of information. Another reason could be that they are more exposed to health risks. Additionally, the social and health services are socially selective (Klein, 2002).

The KiGGS Study (2007) of the Robert-Koch Institute has further enhanced our knowledge on the influence of social status on the health of youth. Alongside the findings mentioned above, it also reports other influences of social status such as the frequency of eating disorders, the subjective perception of own health or the exposure of girls and boys to violence.

The KiGGS data have also been analysed in terms of parents' low income and their level of education. Results show that children and teenagers from low-income families have severe health deficits in several fields. Whereas one-half of the parents of the highest income group consider the health of their 3–10-year-old children to be "very good", only one-third of parents with lowest income say the same. The pattern is similar for 11–17-year-olds. Differences in income also impact on the frequency of mental health problems. Parents from the lowest income group say that about 18% of their 3–10-year-old and 14% of their 11–17-year-old children have behaviour problems. In the highest income group, only 5% of the same age groups are in this situation.

The RKI experts also identify an effect of income on overweight/obesity and sport activities. The biggest differences are observed between girls from 11 to 17 years of age. In this age group, girls from the lowest income group are, at 26.4%, almost twice as likely to be overweight or adipose as girls from high income groups, and only 20% of the 3–10-year-olds coming from the lowest income group belong to a sports club compared to more than 50% of the same age group with a higher income level (BZgA and RKI, 2008).

Economic poverty or—to use a different terminology—low economic capital in combination with low "education capital", "social capital" and "cultural capital", which means low expertise, lack of behavioural skills, poor social networks, little free time, unhealthy working and living conditions and poor health supply lead to health inequality (Schmidt, 2008).

6 Child Poverty and Education

The burden of poverty determines not only the health biography but also the course of education. Language acquisition or perceptual development are affected and thereby influence the ability to learn (i.e. reading) and/or lead to behavioural problems making poor girls and boys already inferior to others of their age group when starting school, and also unable to draw on resources from their milieu.

In three consecutive studies, the *"Kinderpanel"* (child panel) of the *Deutsche Jugendinstitut* (German Youth Institute) has confirmed that continuing poverty as well as the subjective experience of impoverishment influence school performance by, for example, leading to reading problems. Additionally the well-being of children is affected by the pronounced stress of considerable variations in the economic situation of the family while it remains poor (Beisenherz, 2007).

Even at a very early age, social origins play a role in early child education, and unequal education opportunities already manifest at the age of 3. Children from parents with low educational level as well as immigrant children are less likely to attend Kindergarten than non-immigrant children or children from families with a higher educational background (Konsortium Bildungsberichterstattung, 2006). At the transition from primary to secondary school at the age of 10, it is more difficult for pupils from lower social layers to not only enter higher qualifying schools but also to stay in them (Statistisches Bundesamt, 2006).

Programme for International Student Assessment (PISA) studies regularly certify the lack of permeability and the education disadvantage for young migrants and socially disadvantaged youth in general. This leads to few opportunities for them to gain their own life perspective and lift themselves out of poverty. In many cases, family income is the decisive predictor of school performance. The AWO-ISS study has confirmed that children of poor parents—even when they have a good educational level—are less successful in terms of good grades and successful transition to secondary school compared to the students who are not poor (Holz, Richter, Wüstendörfer & Giering, 2005). The study has also shown that the ages at which a child enters Kindergarten and transfers to primary school depend on the financial resources of the parents. Children from socially disadvantaged families often enter Kindergarten only 1 year before school starts, and only 69% of these children enter primary school at the regular age compared to 88% of other children.

We find similar results in international studies showing that economic poverty not only has a massive impact on the course of education but also increases the risk of not completing more than basic, lower-level secondary school education (the German *Hauptschule*). Often, this does not even depend on factors such as social background or family atmosphere. It is particularly interesting to see that poverty has a stronger impact on academic performance development in school than cognitive development when compared to children from higher status groups. The backlog already starts at the beginning of the educational course (Groh-Sandberg and Grundmann 2006).

7 Social Resources, Networks and Social Integration

Social support is seen as an important variable in coping with daily life. However, when a child or family's socioeconomic status is in decline, the quality and frequency of social contacts usually decreases as well and, with this, the available support. Accordingly, the social networks of disadvantaged persons are considerably smaller and usually locally limited compared to those of non-disadvantaged groups. The consequences have been disclosed in several studies: less leisure activities for the children, fewer contacts and offers of support for poor mothers, fewer chances of contacting peers and building friendships for girls and boys with migration backgrounds and many more. Correspondingly, this leads not only to less participation in society but also triggers negative effects on health (Beauftragte der Bundesregierung für Migration & Flüchtlinge und Integration, 2007; Hurrelmann & Andresen, 2007; Hurrelmann et al., 2003; Richter, 2000; Richter & Wächter, 2009).

8 Lack of Jobs and Education

The Joint Report on Social Protection and Social Inclusion 2009 of the European Commission has complained about the inequalities that hinder peoples' chances in life in Europe and in Germany (Commission of the European Communities, 2009). It points out that children face a higher risk of poverty and social exclusion, and that we therefore need strategies combining adequate income support with quality jobs for parents and the provision of necessary services. The Joint Report also confirms persisting inequalities in health status between different socioeconomic groups and different regions and underlines how evidence shows a clear correlation between bad health and poverty, unemployment and low education.

The report notes that most of the EU-27 regard preschool education as fundamental—both as a *key element* in levelling socioeconomic disadvantages and as a means to facilitate work/family life reconciliation. They also consider it highly important to ensure high-quality standards in schools, to fight early school leaving and to improve access to education for certain groups.

Last year's OECD study criticised the dramatic increase in inequality in Germany. For 2007, SOEP shows a rising number of people in low-income jobs, and that even full-time jobs can lead to precarious wage situations. Between 1995 and 2006, low-income jobs lost 14% in terms of real income. Although this trend already started at the beginning of the 1990s, there has been a rapid growth in inequality of available income especially since 2000. SOEP data confirm that despite full-time employment of one parent, every tenth child remains in poverty (Strengmann-Kuhn, 2006). The burden on families needs to be reduced, especially in the lower-income group.

Measures to reduce unemployment are of the utmost importance. The most effective tool against child poverty is employment for the parents—employment in quality jobs that are well-paid, as the Joint Report has pointed out recently (Commission of the European Communities, 2009). However, this is at risk of remaining an ineffective slogan when no jobs are available and, as mentioned above, even full-time jobs can lead to precarious wage situations. Political strategies have to be combined with action; that is, labour market policy has to be combined with family policy for all families. Currently, it corresponds to "middle-class families". Single parents or "low-income families" need more. Their situation is marked by lack of money and lack of support. A diverse and high-quality provision of child-care, meaning care for toddlers, kindergartens and all-day schooling does not yet belong to daily routine in Germany.

The problem partly depends on the lack of early education in Germany. Today, opportunities for development and education greatly depend on family background. Even the European target of care facilities for 90% of all children from 3 years on is only barely reached by Germany (in 2007: Federal State (total Germany) 89.3%, western Germany 88.4%, eastern Germany 94.1%; both excluding Berlin). It is even more difficult when it comes to the under-3s. Childcare provision for under-3s is available for only 10% of children in western Germany. Early education services in Germany need to be extended enormously.

The disadvantage in education is also a result of a lack of financial support for the family to pay for midday meals, fees and working materials for daily schooling and day-care facilities. It is also insufficiently clear how a balanced diet can be ensured under Hartz IV conditions.

9 Social and Economic Policy for Children

The social security systems need to be adapted to reality. There is a major undesirable trend in the financial and distribution system when it comes to day-care facilities, associations (sports, culture, leisure time), public transport, private tuition, school materials and so forth. For Germany, it is a fact that social security (under SGB II/SGB XII) has clearly worsened since the introduction of Hartz IV. We see a growing social inequality that demands urgent action. Findings reported above show that reciprocal influences between education opportunities, health opportunities and child poverty cumulate when disadvantage persists over the life course, and that these continuously affect health and life opportunities. Overall, it must be borne in mind that a person's poverty is primarily a result of societal processes and only secondarily a result of personal failure or personal behaviour. Poverty is a genuine part of a market economy and its distribution mechanisms. Individual failure plays a rather subordinate role in this framework, although it can also contribute to a higher general poverty risk.

An effective policy to ensure a "good childhood" has to aim at preventing poverty and promoting education and health opportunities as well as social integration. For poor children, this currently means improving access—especially access to education and to health services as well as improvements in covering material needs. When we look at child poverty, we have to assess the conditions of growing up in poverty and how growing up in well-being can be assured. Table 1 presents a scheme for analysing which measures are necessary.

What is certain is that it is not just the parents who should be held responsible for this. Within the framework of a new understanding of public responsibility, this has to be a joint task (12. Kinder- und Jugendbericht 2005; 13. Kinder- und Jugendbericht 2009). And this has to be brought into effect on a local level—in the children's surroundings—including extensive and high-quality services in the immediate environment that secure basic provision for *all* children. It is the public authorities that are mainly in charge of assuring this. The national government, the individual states and the municipalities are responsible for offering a framework that may even out the regional disparities, without leaving it to the resources of the municipalities alone.

A public commitment for *all* children can involve three different approaches:

1. Indirect, through measures to help the families/parents that address the labour market, health system, reconciliation of family and job as well as social security.
2. Indirect, through measures addressing the social surroundings, that is, urban development, neighbourhood development, special activities in socially disadvantaged areas, healthy neighbourhoods, healthy cities, setting-orientated arrangements of health promotion.
3. Direct, through measures adapted to children providing early interventions, crèche facilities, day-care facilities, free teaching materials, improved transitions in the education system, promotion of high-quality all-day schools, access to health care and health check-ups, free access to sports clubs, swimming pools and music schools as well as free public transport (Butterwegge, 2009; Holz, 2008; Richter, 2008).

10 Health Policy for Poor Children

The WHO (1986) stresses the importance of the environment when aiming to promote health. This perception leads to the strategy of action *in settings*—a very promising approach, especially when trying to reach the socially disadvantaged. Because it is seen as vital to follow this approach towards quality in health promotion for socially disadvantaged persons, it has been included in the "*Leitfaden Prävention*" (prevention guideline) of the Federal health insurance companies. This guideline explicitly names kindergartens, schools and districts as deserving support. It describes the targets, principles and implementation of health promotion within settings. In accordance with the Ottawa Charter, the guideline names the combination of measures aimed at surroundings and behaviour. Health insurance companies expect the proposed measures to be embedded in networks and health promotion strategies that span political fields. For promotion in schools, this means, for example, that other responsible stakeholders (education providers, child and youth services) also integrate health promotion as a guiding model and orientation. These processes will be subjected to quality control and comply with existing criteria. They have been developed by a working group of experts from a wide range of fields (scientists, practitioners, NGOs etc.) and have found broad approval.

The Joint Report on Social Protection and Social Inclusion 2009 points out that although promotion and health prevention are considered to be the preferred way to improve health, they receive relatively low funding to cover the objectives they are supposed to meet (Commission of the European Communities, 2009). Germany, in particular, spends a lot of money on health care, especially medical and clinical treatment. The total amount is 260 billion Euros per year. Expenditure for health promotion and prevention is included in this and specified under § 20 SGB V (article 20 of the Social Security Statute Book): "These services for primary prevention shall improve the general status of health and contribute in particular to the mitigation of socially induced inequality in health opportunities".

But today, this is little more than rhetoric. Germany spent 350 million Euros on this in 2007. This equals 4.30 Euros per person. However, most of this spending was on an individual level and given for courses like back exercise programmes. Moreover, it is spent without us knowing whether the money is being applied effectively. Children only represent 4% of the patients in these programmes, although they represent 14% of all people insured. And these services are usually not used at all by those who are socially disadvantaged. In 2008, the health insurance scheme published a prevention report documenting its activities in settings on more than 35 pages. However this is not followed up and is simply paying lip service. The sum invested in primary prevention especially dedicated to settings amounted to only 0.35 cents per person in 2007.

11 Policy for Best Practice

Policy strategies need to be linked to practice in order to be effective. In the field of health promotion for the socially disadvantaged, there are several important demands. Above all, we have to ensure that those existing arrangements that work are adapted to the target group of disadvantaged children. What is essential in this field is access for *all* children. Their opportunities have to be improved by targeted encouragement. The atmosphere in schools and classes has to be promoted. Training of teachers and Kindergarten teachers has to be improved, too, and standards in equipment need to be reassessed.

We have to act on settings!

Today, we know that if we want to reach the target group—disadvantaged people—we have to apply a wide range of methods within settings such as districts, neighbourhoods, kindergartens and schools. We need, for example, health promotion with an emphasis on the individual as well as on community capacity building and empowerment. We need to perceive the setting orientation as both a behaviour orientation *and* an orientation towards surroundings or basic conditions, and we need to invest in the children's environment.

We need cooperation instead of competition!

We need intersectional cooperation. But what are we doing today? We invest in social security systems—to enable people to cope with *single* life-risks—while making hardly any integrated investment into the child's environment. What is missing is target-group-oriented health concepts and sustainable investment in education. The German education system is above all selective and demanding, not supportive and integrative.

We need quality in this process!

Quality needs to be assessed with criteria such as the realization of participation, empowerment, capacity building and low barrier methods. Only success in participation, including different methods of participation can improve access to common arrangements and measures for disadvantaged people. Participation in this way includes

- Formulation of desires, needs and criticism
- Participation in decisions
- Participation in making rules
- Active inclusion of all persons affected in the planning, implementation and evaluation of services (Block, von Unger & Wright, 2009)

Other quality criteria such as capacity building have already been mentioned. We need experiences in intersectional action, in cooperation between the health, education, youth welfare service and community work sectors as well. We need to know more about what the obstacles are and what the advantages are. And we must not forget that when quality is required, it has to be paid for. This also includes the costs of evaluating the measures.

We know this. We do not have a knowledge deficit, but an action deficit. We need more. Although the different reports mentioned above stress the great importance of action, long-term strategies to prevent and tackle social exclusion are missing. However, the access and use of these services for girls and boys affected by poverty will shape the future of our society.

References

3. Armuts- und Reichtumsbericht der Bundesregierung (2008). *Lebenslagen in Deutschland.* Bonn/Berlin: BMAS.
12. Kinder- und Jugendbericht. (2005). *Bildung, Betreuung und Erziehung vor und neben der Schule. Bericht über die Lebenssituation junger Menschen und die Leistungen der Kinder- und Jugendhilfe in Deutschland.* Accessed September 30, 2009, from http://www.bmfsfj.de/doku/kjb/data/haupt.html
13. Kinder- und Jugendbericht. (2009). *Bericht über gesundheitsbezogene Prävention und Gesundheitsförderung in der Kinder- und Jugendhilfe. Bericht über die Lebenssituation junger Menschen und die Leistungen der Kinder- und Jugendhilfe in Deutschland.* Berlin, Germany: Deutscher Bundestag, Drucksache 16/12860.
Adamy, W. (2008). *Hohes Verarmungsrisiko Jugendlicher.* Accessed May 13, 2009, from http://bildungsklick.de/datei-archiv/50648/studie_verarmungsrisiko_jugend.pdf
Beauftragte der Bundesregierung für Migration, Flüchtlinge und Integration. (2007). 7. *Bericht der Beauftragten der Bundesregierung für Migration, Flüchtlinge und Integration über die Lage der Ausländerinnen und Ausländer in Deutschland.* Berlin, Germany.
Beck, I. (2002). Die Lebenslagen von Kindern und Jugendlichen mit Behinderung und ihrer Familien in Deutschland: Soziale und strukturelle Dimensionen. In Sachverständigenkommission 11. Kinder- und Jugendbericht (Ed.), *Gesundheit und Behinderung im Leben von Kindern und Jugendlichen* (pp. 175–315). Munich.
Beisenherz, G. H. (2007). Wohlbefinden und Schulleistung von Kindern armer Familien. In C. Alt (Ed.), *Kinderleben – Start in die Grundschule Bd. 3: Ergebnisse aus der zweiten Welle des Kinderpanels.* Wiesbaden: VS-Verlag für Sozialwissenschaften.
Bildungsberichterstattung, Ko. nsortium (2006). *Bildung in Deutschland.* Gütersloh: Bertelsmann.
Block, M., von Unger, H., & Wright, M. T. (2009). Partizipation von Kindern als Schlüssel der Gesundheitsförderung. Ein Beitrag zur Qualität in der Armutsprävention? In C. Butterwegge (Ed.), *Armut in einem reichem Land. Wie das Problem verharmlost und verdrängt wird.* Frankfurt a. M.: Campus.
Statistisches Bundesamt. (2006). *Statistisches Jahrbuch für die Bundesrepublik Deutschland 2006.* Accessed March 12, 2009, from http://www-ec.destatis.de/csp/shop/sfg/bpm.html.cms.cBroker.cls?cmspath=struktur,vollanzeige.csp&ID=1019209

Butterwegge Ch. (2009). Armut in einem reichen Land. Wie das Problem verharmlost und verdrängt wird. Frankfurt a. M.: Campus Verlag.

BZgA and RKI. (2008). *Erkennen – Bewerten – Handeln: Zur Gesundheit von Kindern und Jugendlichen in Deutschland*. Berlin.

Commission of the European Communities. (2009). *Joint report on social protection and social inclusion*. Brussels, Belgium.

Corak, M., Fertig, M., & Tamm, M. (2005). *A portrait of child poverty in Germany*. (Discussion Papers No. 26). Essen, Germany: RWI.

Fertig, M. & M. Tamm (2007). Kinderarmut im internationalen Vergleich. In: Deutsches Kinderhilfswerk (ed.), *Kinderreport Deutschland 2007*, Freiburg: Velber.

Fertig, M. & M. Tamm (2008). Die Verweildauer von Kindern in prekären Lebenslagen. In: H. Bertram (ed.), *Mittelmaß für Kinder – Der UNICEF-Bericht zur Lage der Kinder in Deutschland*, München: Verlag C. H. Beck, 152–166.

Groh-Samberg, O., & Grundmann, M. (2006). Soziale Ungleichheit im Kindes- und Jugendalter. *Aus Politik und Zeitgeschichte*, 26, 11–24.

Hock, B., Holz, G., Simmedinger, R., & Wüstendörfer, W. (1999). *Gute Kindheit – Schlechte Kindheit? Armut und Zukunftschancen von Kindern und Jugendlichen in Deutschland*. Frankfurt a. M.: ISS-Aktuell.

Holz, G. (2008). Institutionelle Strukturen und ihre Rolle für die Verfestigung von Kinderarmut. In AGF – Arbeitsgemeinschaft der deutschen Familienorganisationen (Ed.), *Kinderarmut – eine strukturelle Herausforderung* (pp. 20–37). Berlin. http://www.ag-familie.de/Tagungen.html. Accessed October 1, 2009.

Holz, G., Richter, A., Wüstendörfer, W., & Giering, D. (2005). *Zukunftschancen für Kinder!? – Wirkung von Armut bis zum Ende der Grundschulzeit*. Endbericht der 3. AWO-ISS-Studie im Auftrag der Arbeiterwohlfahrt Bundesverband e.V. Frankfurt a. M.: ISS-Aktuell.

Hurrelmann, K., & Andresen, S. (2007). *Kinder in Deutschland 2007*. 1. World Vision Kinderstudie. Frankfurt: Fischer.

Hurrelmann, K., Klocke, A., Melzer, W., & Ravens-Sieberer, U. (2003). WHO-Jugendgesundheitssurvey – Konzept und ausgewählte Ergebnisse für die Bundesrepublik Deutschland. *Erziehungswissenschaft*, 27, 79–108.

KiGGS. (2008). *Kinder- und Jugendgesundheitssurvey 2003–2006 – Kinder und Jugendliche mit Migrationshintergrund in Deutschland. Beiträge zur Gesundheitsberichterstattung des Bundes*. Berlin, Germany.

Klein, G. (2002). *Frühförderung für Kinder mit psychosozialen Risiken*. Stuttgart: Kohlhammer.

Lampert, T., Kroll, L. E., & Dunkelberg, A. (2007). Soziale Ungleichheit der Lebenserwartung in Deutschland. *Aus Politik und Zeitgeschichte*, 42, 11–18.

Mielk, A. (2000). Armut macht krank – immer noch. *Gesundheit und Gesellschaft*, 6, 32–37.

Mielk, A. (2004). Armut als Krankheitsrisiko. Impulse 43: Chronisch krank – chronisch arm? *Newsletter zur Gesundheitsförderung*, 2, 5–6.

Mielk, A. (2008, June). *Zwischen Wunsch und Wirklichkeit – bedarfsgerechte Versorgung für Alle*. Unpublished lecture given at the International Symposium Health Inequalities III, Bielefeld, Germany.

OECD. (2008). *Growing unequal? Income distribution and poverty in OECD-countries*. Paris: Author.

Richter, A. (2000). *Wie erleben und bewältigen Kinder Armut? Eine qualitative Studie über die Belastungen aus Unterversorgungslagen und ihre Bewältigung aus subjektiver Sicht von Grundschulkindern einer ländlichen Region*. Aachen: Shaker.

Richter, A. (2008). Armut und Resilienz – Was stärkt arme Kinder? *Verhaltenstherapie und psychosoziale Praxis*, 40(3), 249–268.

Richter, A., Holz, G., & Altgeld, T. (2004). *Gesund in allen Lebenslagen. Förderung von Gesundheitspotentialen bei sozial benachteiligten Kindern im Elementarbereich*. Frankfurt a. M.: ISS-Aktuell.

Richter, A., & Wächter, M. (2009). *Zum Zusammenhang von Nachbarschaft und Gesundheit*. Accessed September 30, 2009, from http://www.bzga.de/bigpix.php?id= e24866761688775ef13bf91ec6876ed5&w=514&h&=700

Rosenbrock, R. (2004). *Primäre Prävention zur Verminderung sozial bedingter Ungleichheit von Gesundheitschancen. 13 Befunde und Empfehlungen*. Essen: BKK Bundesverband.

Schäfer, C. (2008). Anhaltende Verteilungsdramatik – WSI-Verteilungsbericht 2008. *WSI Mitteilungen, 11*, 12, 587–596.

Schlack, H. G. (2003). Socially underprivileged children: A challenge for communal health care. *Gesundheitswesen, 65*, 671–675.

Schmidt, B. (2008). *Eigenverantwortung haben immer die Anderen. Der Verantwortungsdiskurs im Gesundheitswesen*. Bern: Huber.

Strengmann-Kuhn, W. (2006). Vermeidung von Kinderarmut in Deutschland durch finanzielle Leistungen. *Zeitschrift für Sozialreform/ Journal of Social Policy Research, 52*(4), 439–466.

Weiß, H. (2000). *Frühförderung mit Kindern und Familien in Armutslagen*. Munich: Reinhardt.

WHO (1986) Ottawa Charter for Health Promotion. WHO/HPR/HEP/95.1,Geneva.

Well-Being of Children in Turkey

Didem Gürses

1 Introduction

A child growing up without access to the economic, physical and environmental resources needed for survival and development is experiencing poverty. Child poverty covers both the material and nonmaterial deprivation experienced by many children and young people. It is a multidimensional concept encompassing nutritional, educational and health-related needs as well as more subjective factors such as security, affection and other emotional development needs. As childhood is the most vital period in an individual's mental, physical and social development, deprivation during this life phase in terms of nutrition, health care, affection and security—even for short periods of time—can have long-term and irreversible consequences.

Child poverty, being a problem in both poor and rich countries, still prevails throughout the world. The 2005 review of child poverty in rich countries from the UNICEF Innocenti Research Centre indicates that it has risen in 17 out of 24 OECD nations over the last decade (UNICEF-IRC, 2005, p. 4).

Although Turkey was hit by a severe financial crisis in February 2001, the impacts of which were very harsh and extensive, the economy managed to recover after 2002. For the last 5 years, Turkey has been growing consistently and is now accepted as an upper-middle income country and a dynamic emerging market. However, disparities between regions and genders are still large, and the country faces significant inequalities in income distribution. Additionally, gender disparities and variations among geographical regions and social groups are observed in terms of health, education and political representation. Education continues to be a major factor underlying gender disparity; there is still a gap in literacy between males and females. Moreover, the impacts of economic policies implemented after the 1980s and the effects of the military dispute during the 1990s in the south eastern parts of

D. Gürses (✉)
Department of Humanities and Social Sciences, Yildiz Technical University, 34210 Esenler, Istanbul, Turkey
e-mail: dgurses@yildiz.edu.tr

S. Andresen et al. (eds.), *Children and the Good Life*, Children's Well-Being: Indicators and Research 4, DOI 10.1007/978-90-481-9219-9_13, © Springer Science+Business Media B.V. 2010

the country are reflected deeply in the social and economic structure. As a result of these developments, the incidence of poverty has begun to increase since the 1990s and has become more visible, especially in the cities. This chapter aims to examine the situation of children in Turkey. The focus will be on children, but as they are dependent on their parents and caregivers, it will also analyse the situation of the family and the social environment that impact directly on the children's well-being. The situation of children in the country will be considered in terms of maternal and child health, education and child labour. It starts with an overview of poverty in Turkey in general followed by the situation of children in particular. The next section assesses Turkish social policy strategies that aim to have a positive impact on children's well-being and evaluates the social protection mechanisms. The chapter concludes with a summary and discussion of the findings, before pointing to areas requiring reform.

2 Manifestation of Poverty in Contemporary Turkey

Turkey has been experiencing radical socioeconomic transformations over the last three decades. Starting in the 1980s, its economic policy has been largely shaped by changes away from an import-substituting industrialization model towards a more outward looking and market-oriented strategy of integration in the global economy. This fundamental transition may be identified with different dimensions of a complex but unitary phenomenon: deindustrialization, post-Fordism and globalization. Their impact manifested in agricultural reforms, a decrease in employment opportunities in the formal manufacturing sector and/or state-owned enterprises as well as an informalization of the labour market. The end result of the informalization of the labour market has been declining chances for an informal sector employee to find work in the formal sector. Informal jobs not only imply lack of access to social security provisions but also mean the absence of a reliable work contract (Bugra and Keyder, 2005, p. 26; Keyder, 2005, p. 127).

The Turkish economy faced serious crises in 1994, 1998–1999 and 2000–2001, each of which was followed by a complete collapse of the economy that could only be stabilized after IMF intervention (Demir, 2004, p. 853). The outcomes of these crises have been drastic regressions in real income for the working masses, decreases in employment opportunities and a worsening of income shares for the poorest groups. Moreover, the military conflict during the 1990s caused the poorest segments of the eastern and the south eastern regions to migrate to the big cities. As a result of these developments, the incidence of poverty increased in both urban and rural regions of the country during the late 1990s—deeply affecting the most vulnerable segments, the women and the children.

Even though absolute poverty is low in Turkey, at about 0.74%, economic vulnerability is quite high for a middle-income country. It affects about one-fifth (17.81%) of the population and is concentrated mostly in the south-eastern and eastern regions (Turkstat, 2006). The findings of Turkstat reveal that Turkey has made considerable progress since the financial crisis of 2001. In 2002, approximately one-third of the population (29.6%) was economically vulnerable (Turkstat, 2007a). In 2006, this had dropped to 17.8%. Although a significant decrease, the current situation implies that 4.2 million urban and 8.7 million rural, that is, a total of 12.9 million people, still have no sufficient means to obtain food, clothing and shelter in the country (Turkstat, 2006).

Poverty in Turkey is strongly linked to the nature and form of employment, educational attainment, household size and number of children, type of housing and the residential area. The disparities between urban and rural regions are reflected deeply in the incidence of poverty. A poverty rate of 9.3% in the urban regions rises to 31.9% in rural areas.

Illiterate household heads represent 10.12% of the Turkish population but account for 33.71% of the poor households. As the education of the person increases, poverty incidence drops dramatically. While poverty incidence is 14.19% among primary school graduates, it drops to 5.20% among high school graduates (Turkstat, 2006).

Labour market status is another important correlate of poverty. The risk of poverty is highest (31.98%) for households in which the head is an unpaid family worker. Households of unpaid family workers are even more vulnerable to poverty than the unemployed. Poverty in Turkey is especially a threat for families with many children. In terms of household size, the rate of poverty for families with one child is 11%, whereas it rises to 36.3% for families with three children.

The analysis of poverty risk in relation to age structure reveals that the 0–15 age group faces the highest risk of poverty. About one-third of this age group experiences poverty whereas the proportion drops to 21% in the age group of over–65s (Buğra & Keyder, no date, p. 52).

Various studies have found that the eastern and south-eastern parts of the country have the highest poverty rates. Dumanlı reports that 43.8% of the people living in these regions experience poverty. Central Anatolia follows this region at 26.3% (Dumanlı, 1996, p. 125, p. 162, p. 168). In a different approach, Akder has used aggregated and geographical data at the level of administrative districts based on the human development (HD) index to conclude that low human development is rather a widespread rural phenomenon, whereas high-level human development is very sparse in Turkey. When applying the human development approach to the whole country, he found that 14% of all Turkish districts are classified as having low HD indices, and low human development dominates particularly the south-eastern and east Anatolian regions (Akder, 2000, pp. 32–33). The report prepared by the World Bank based on 1987 and 1994 HICES data indicates that Turkey is a country with large and entrenched inequalities. Income differentials across regions and social groups are widespread and persistent. When measured by the Gini coefficient, inequality in Turkey is close to the levels observed in some highly polarized economies such as Peru or Russia (World Bank, 2000, p. 19).

According to the poverty research carried out under the auspices of the United Nations Development Programme (UNDP), it appears that there is an increase in "new poverty" in Turkey—poverty that is long term and not easily remedied by access to traditional support networks such as family and friends. Social groups affected by the new poverty perceive existing conditions as being more or less permanent and no longer see any solutions to their problems (Buğra & Keyder, 2003, p. 9). The study of the World Bank (WB)—conducted in the summer of 2001 to learn about the social impact of the financial crises—has also reached similar conclusions. The coping mechanisms of the poor, such as assistance from traditional channels, especially relying on the relatives for assistance in kind or cash, have come under stress and have dropped in size (World Bank, 2003, p. 45). The findings of both surveys (Buğra & Keyder, 2003; World Bank, 2003) have reached the same conclusion: People in general felt they were worse off and have lost hope for the future.

An examination of Turkey's position in the human development continuum shows that the country's overall HD performance has been somewhat unpredictable and at times even disappointing. Turkey has made significant improvements in certain spheres, such as infant mortality and was doing quite well during the 1990s. If the upward trend of the 1990s had continued, Turkey could have become one of the "high development countries". Unfortunately, that upward trend did not continue; on the contrary, Turkey lost considerable altitude with respect to its relative HD index rank (UNDP, 2004, p. 11). Moreover international comparisons show that some countries with lower GDP per capita have performed better in relation to literacy and school enrolment than Turkey, which means that Turkey has not been successful in converting her economic growth into individual's quality of life.

Additionally, gender disparities and variations among geographic regions and social groups can be observed in terms of health, education, employment and political representation. Education continues to be a major factor underlying gender disparity; there is still a gap in literacy between males (95.3%) and females (79.9%). The National Human Development Report (NHDR) of Turkey for 2004 reports the male and female HD index by province. High male human development is present in about two-thirds of the country, largely in the east, centre and southwest, whereas high female human development is concentrated in the more urbanized areas and in western parts of the country. In general, women have lower HD values than men. The male-female HD difference is largest in the province of Diyarbakir, in the southeast of Turkey (http://hdr.undp.org/en/reports nationalreports/europethecis/turkey-/turkey_2004_en.pdf).

In Turkey, women were given suffrage in 1933. However, women were elected to only 50 out of the 550 (9.1%) seats in parliament in the 2007 elections. Moreover, female labour participation in the country is still low, with women comprising less than 25% of the registered workforce (Turkstat, 2007). The Gender Empowerment Measure (GEM) for the year 2005, a global indicator of women's economic and political participation, decision making and level of control over economic resources, ranks Turkey in 76th place, which is not fitting for any modern and middle-income society. Although Turkey has made improvements in women's living standards over the last 25 years, almost all social indicators tend to be worse for women than for men, and generally Turkey does worse on gender indicators than comparable middle-income countries.

3 The Situation of Children in Turkey

In Turkey, two decades of market-led economic growth has not been successful in reducing poverty in general. The economic and social policies of recent years have caused a major transformation in the social structure of the country. The role of the state in the economy has been modified, and formal employment opportunities in both the public and private sector have become limited. Liberalization policies implemented since the 1980s included such measures as restricting public expenditure, and this has impacted negatively on the poorest segments of the society whose asset bases are the most limited. These recent developments caused an increase in poverty in the late 1990s, and children of the poorest families have been deeply affected. In Turkey, about one-third of the under-15s are experiencing poverty, and this increases to 49.3% in the rural regions (Turkstat, 2006). Children most at risk of poverty include those who are born into large families with uneducated or scarcely educated parents, whose parents have recently migrated to the cities, whose parents are unemployed or work in informal jobs with no regular income, and who live in rural and mostly eastern and south-eastern regions of the country.

As maternal and child health, education and child labour are the three most important factors influencing the well-being of children, the situation of children will be analysed in relation to these variables. With 1.5 million births each year, Turkey has the highest number of newborns in Europe. Infant and maternal mortality rates are high compared to other middle-income countries and among the highest in Europe. Although a great deal has been done to reduce child mortality rates during the last 25 years, there is still room for improvement. The TDHS (Turkish Demographic and Health Survey) for 2003 reveals that infant and under-5 mortality rates are still 40% higher than the national average in the north and eastern regions. Levels of malnutrition also follow the pattern of urban/rural inequality: The stunted growth rate for under-5s is recorded as 9% in urban areas, 18% in rural areas, 5% in the west and 23% in the east (TDHS, 2005, p. 151).

Turkey has achieved a dramatic reduction in infant mortality rates (IMR) from 150 per 1,000 live births in 1970 to 29 per 1,000 in 2003. Although a remarkable success, the rate is still too high in comparison to countries with similar income levels and HD index rankings. The Human Development Reports reveal that some countries with substantially lower HD index rankings than Turkey have performed better in reducing infant mortality rates. Moreover, there is much variation in urban/rural and western/eastern parts of the country in relation to infant and child mortality rates. For urban areas, IMR is 23 per 1,000 live births; whereas in the rural areas, it rises to 39 per 1,000. IMR is 22 per 1,000 in the western parts and it rises to 41 per 1,000 in the eastern parts of the country (TDHS, 2005, p. 113).

Provision of health and educational services at the regional level, especially in the eastern and south-eastern regions of the country, is hindered by problems of access and security. Although there have been steady improvements in relation to child and maternal health, the issue still continues to be marked by serious problems due to the persistence of broad geographical, economic and cultural disparities at the national level.

Education still continues to be a serious issue for Turkey. Although governments have struggled to increase the adult literacy rate since the foundation of the republic, there is still room for improvement. In 2006, a total of 20% of women and 4% of men were illiterate and the overall literacy rate for the country was 88.1% (Turkstat, 2006). Despite remarkable progress, gender equality in education has not been achieved, and women continue to lag behind men on almost all indicators (Acar, 2003, p. 33).

The Basic Education Law adopted in August 1997 mandated 8 years of compulsory education, aiming to expand opportunities for all children to attend grades 1 through 8 and to increase the quality of education. The government's investments in the Basic Education programme yielded a dramatic increase in education coverage; net enrolment in grades 1 through 8 rose from 81 to 90% (Hoşgör, 2005, p. 90).

Despite the rapid expansion in primary school enrolment and the significant improvements in the access of the poor and of girls to school, gender and poverty gaps in education continue to affect Turkey's education indicators. Aggregate education statistics indicate that roughly 10% of Turkish children aged 6–14 years are not enrolled in basic education. Large shares of this population belong to two groups: girls and the poor (Mete, 2005, p. 101).

With regard to non-compulsory schooling, the situation is worse. Turkey has one of the lowest preschool education coverage among all lower-middle-income countries. Less than 14% of children aged 4–6 years were enrolled in preschool in 2003, whereas the average enrolment rate for middle-income countries is 36% (Kaytaz, 2005, p. 96).

Furthermore, access to secondary school continues to be limited by the availability of school places, especially in rural areas, as well as family choices. Gender and poverty gaps are greater at the level of secondary education: One in three high-school-aged girls is not attending school, compared to only one in 10 boys. This is the largest gender gap among EU member and candidate countries. The situation in the southeast where, in 2003, only 14% of girls were attending secondary school, is even more frustrating (World Bank, 2005, p. 4).

In general, Turkey has increased educational achievement over the last 40 years, as measured by all indicators, in spite of political and economic instability. In order to develop education to meet Europe averages, targeted strategies to increase enrolment rates should be initiated at all education levels especially in the four important regions of East Black Sea, North Eastern Anatolia, South Eastern Anatolia and East Anatolia. The education system should also be evaluated according to the needs of the country and its prospects for EU membership (Hoşgör, 2005, p. 94).

Child poverty is closely related to child labour and removal of children from school. The children of poor families are obliged to work in unhealthy and unsafe conditions. This is a perfect example of how the burden of poverty impacts on children in terms of deprivation from education. The problem of child labour is highlighted in the Joint Inclusion Memorandum prepared by the Ministry of Labour and Social Security (Buğra & Keyder, no date, p. 12).

In 1992, Turkey was one of the first six countries to undertake direct action to fight child labour through the International Program on the Elimination of Child

(IPEC) Labour. The project has reached 50,000 children, and 60% of them have been withdrawn from work and placed in school. As a result, Turkey's efforts are now accepted as good practice in the fight against child labour. Although great progress has been achieved, there are still serious problems to be solved. According to the statistics for the year 2000, 11.3% of the 12–14 age group is still working and the percentage of children not attending school among the compulsory school age group is still high.

4 Social Protection Mechanisms

The Social Assistance and Solidarity Fund (SASF) is the main public institution in the field of poverty alleviation in the country. Established in 1986, the fund was set up to help people in a state of poverty and to take measures to enforce social justice by ensuring fair distribution of income. Especially since the mid-1990s, the fund has distributed a non-negligible amount of resources to provide health and education support as well as to satisfy the urgent needs of those in extreme poverty, mostly through in-kind transfers of fuel or food.

In 1992, the Government launched a "Green Card Program" to provide health care services to poor people who are not covered by any of the existing social security systems. Currently, there are about 13 million Green Card holders, and expenditure on their health constitutes the largest item in the budget of SASF. The second largest item in the fund's budget is allocated to students at different levels, including scholarships, provision of school supplies, meals and snacks for school children.

After the 2001 financial crisis, the government started allocating financial resources through the Social Risk Mitigation Project (SRMP) supported by the World Bank. Conditional Cash Transfers (CCT), first adopted under the SRMP, aimed to provide an incentive to the poor to keep their children in school. Through the coordinated work of the Ministry of Health (MoH) and the Ministry of National Education (MoNE), cash transfers are made to the poorest segments of the population in order to provide them with basic health and education services. Expectant mothers and families with children up to 6 years of age receive small amounts of money when they visit health centres for regular check-ups. Another form of payment is made on an educational basis. SASF is providing a conditional cash transfer for poor families who send their children to school with an extra 20% incentive for girls, and this payment is made to the mothers. Since 2003, the number of students benefiting from the CCT has increased.

Implementation of CCT is an important and new phase in Turkey's social policy. Designed to minimize the negative effects of the 2001 financial crisis, these cash transfers address both future and current poverty. By promoting education and health controls, they work as a means of investment in human capital and therefore deal with future poverty. The provision of income, on the other hand, helps the poor to cope with their current poverty. This includes preventing the social exclusion of the poorest segments from society and avoiding the burden of poverty impacting on children in the form of malnutrition and deprivation from education.

Beginning in the 2003 school year, the government started a new measure. In order to prevent school dropouts due to poverty, the Ministry of National Education (MoNE) began to provide free school textbooks to all primary school students. Free textbooks for the secondary school students were also made available in 2006.

Established to provide services to children in need of protection, the Social Services and Child Protection Agency (SHCEK) provides institutional care and family services, child adoption, social assistance, nursery and daily care services for children who are in material or psychological need. Besides children, the agency's responsibilities also include elderly people and women exposed to violence. Targeting a wide range of groups but not having the necessary financial and technical capacity, the institution has failed to outreach the population in need and the services provided remain very poor. For the provision of adequate social assistance to children in need, its institutional and operational capacity should be improved and outreach skills should be developed.

Turkey has ratified the International Conventions on children's and women's rights such as the International Convention on the Rights of the Child (CRC) and the Convention on the Elimination of All Forms of Discrimination against Women (CEDAW). Since the 1990s, Turkey has included in its programs the revision of internal procedures, withdrawal of reservations and the development of policies consistent with international organizations such as the UN, the European Council, ILO, OECD and the European Security and Cooperation conference regarding women and children. The General Directorate for Women's Status and Problems was established in 1990 and since then has been implementing a national programme to enhance women's integration in development, to raise women's social status, to increase their level of education and to enable them to take part in working life and decision making. As part of these efforts, the minimum marriage age for girls was raised from 15 to 17, a juvenile justice system is being established for children and youth, and a new civil code has been introduced giving women equal rights over matrimonial property.

5 Conclusion

As mentioned above, an important segment of the Turkish population, particularly in rural areas, is vulnerable to the threats of poverty. Recent research shows that a new form of poverty in urban areas is also becoming a challenge for policy makers. Inequality cuts across regions, incomes, knowledge, human development and gender. The 2001 Human Development Report underlines the problem of inequality, stating that this could result in inefficiency and trigger social problems such as uncontrolled urbanization, crime and social unrest (UNDP, 2001, p. 3). Findings indicate that a substantial proportion of children are growing up without the resources and services they need to develop into healthy, productive and happy adults. High levels of inequality at various fields of life present significant barriers to children's development.

Although the government has adopted a proactive attitude especially since the 2001 financial crisis, and has introduced new elements into the social assistance system, poverty in general and childhood poverty in particular still continue to be a serious issue on Turkey's agenda. Not only the economic and political structure of the country but also the regional, religious and ethnic features of the population affect and shape the dynamics, extent, dimensions and depth of this problem. Research findings have shown that issues related to gender may operate as significant causes of poverty. Women's and girls' access to education, health services and employment is hindered by gender-related issues that, in turn, add to their vulnerable position in society. It is a well-known fact that household income is not shared evenly; on the contrary, there is a traditional gender bias favouring the boys of the family over girls. Therefore, the policies designed to eradicate child poverty must take into account all these determinants and the social realities of the country.

Turkey has not been successful in developing a coherent and comprehensive national policy to struggle against poverty in general and child poverty in particular. In order to form a social, political, economic and cultural environment enabling every child to have adequate opportunities to achieve his or her full potential, the government has to recognize the uniqueness of childhood poverty with its distinct needs. Being a country in a rapid transformation process, a wide range of economic, political, cultural and social factors leads to childhood poverty. The unpredictable and fluctuating nature of the country's social conditions needs to be taken into account when designing a comprehensive national anti-poverty policy.

One of the main shortcomings of the current Turkish social security system is that it is mainly dependant on holding a formal-sector job. Therefore, it usually fails to reach the poorest segments of the population. However, research has revealed that children most at risk of poverty include the ones whose parents work in informal and casual employment and have no regular income along with those whose parents are either long-term unemployed or underemployed and thereby not covered by any social insurance system. As these groups are the ones most deeply affected by crises and they are the poorest segments of the society, Turkey has to develop systematic interventions and design new and creative mechanisms to reach out to those who cannot be reached through existing formal protective schemes.

The recent financial crises have also shown that Turkey's current data on poverty cannot provide policy makers with reliable and adequate information about the national causes, dynamics, extent, dimension and depth of poverty and especially child poverty. Therefore, the government has to establish a broad database. Qualitative and quantitative techniques must be used in conjunction to arrive at a deeper understanding of poverty (Şenses, 2003, p. 338).

The scattered structure of the social assistance system in the country prevents coordination and cooperation among the existing social assistance institutions. This, in turn, leads to a waste of resources and lack of transparency and accountability. Absence of an efficient flow of information about the social assistance provided and the people benefiting from it may cause duplications, poor targeting and even misuse. This situation has also been acknowledged in the progress report of Turkey's

Integration to the EU. It has been stated that "the existing structures that support social inclusion are scattered and fragmented. There is a lack of coordination, therefore interested public organizations and the other related stakeholders must be activated under an integrated approach" (SPO, 2004, p. 99).

It must be kept in mind that poverty is a multidimensional concept and wears a multitude of faces. It is a very dynamic and complex process with multiple and interacting causes, meanings and manifestations. The policies designed to struggle against poverty and, in particular, child poverty should acknowledge this aspect of the issue. The objective should be to improve children's quality of life and well-being rather than simply to reduce poverty.

In combating child poverty, Turkey should embrace child-focused social policies and especially invest in the capabilities of the children. Access to good quality, accessible and affordable primary health care, primary education and early childhood development programmes are vital for fighting against child poverty. This includes maternal and child health care, preventive and curative health care services, child and mother nutrition and a service provision for children at all ages. It is generally agreed all over the world that, as women are the catalysts of change and advocates of children's rights, adoption of policies that will empower women, such as improvement of employment opportunities for women and achievement of gender equality, will help to accelerate the solution to the problem of child poverty. Accepting the fight against childhood poverty as a political priority and building strategies to improve the situation of the poorest families and their children will function as an indispensable investment for both the present and the future of the country.

References

Acar, F. (2003). Women's education. In World Bank. Poverty Reduction and Economic Management Unit Europe and Central Asia (Ed.), *Bridging the gender gap in Turkey: A milestone towards faster socio-economic development and poverty reduction* (pp. 32–53). Washington, DC: World Bank.

Akder, H. (2000). *Regional development and rural poverty*. İstanbul: TESEV.

Buğra, A., & Keyder, Ç. (2003). *New poverty and the changing welfare regime of Turkey*. Ankara: UNICEF.

Buğra, A., & Keyder, Ç. (2005). *Poverty and social policy in contemporary Turkey*. Report of Bogazici University, Social Policy Forum. Accessed September 28, 2009, from http://www.spf.boun.edu.tr/docs/WP-Bugra-Keyder.pdf

Buğra, A., & Keyder, Ç. (2006). *Social assistance in Turkey: For a policy of minimum income support conditional on socially beneficial activity*. Ankara: UNDP.

Demir, F. (2004). A failure story: Politics and financial liberalization in Turkey, revisiting the revolving door hypothesis. *World Development, 32*(5), 851–869.

Dumanlı, R. (1996). *Yoksulluk ve Türkiye'deki Boyutlar* (Poverty and its dimensions in Turkey). Ankara: DPT Yayınları.

Hoşgör, S. (2005). *Status and trends in education*. Paper commissioned for the Turkey Education Sector Study. Washington, DC: World Bank.

Kaytaz, M. (2005). *A cost-benefit analysis of pre-school education in Turkey*. Paper Commissioned for the Turkey Education Sector Study. Washington, DC: World Bank.

Keyder, Ç. (2005). Globalization and social exclusion in Istanbul. *International Journal of Regional Research, 29*(1), 124–134.

Mete, C. (2005). *Education finance and equity in Turkey*. Paper commissioned for the Turkey Education Sector Study, Washington, DC: World Bank.

SPO. (2004). *Türkiye'nin AB'ne katılım sürecine ilişkin* 2004 *yılı ilerleme raporu ve tavsiye metni* (Progress Report and Recommendation Note on Turkey's EU Accession Process for 2004). Ankara: DPT.

Şenses, F. (2003). *Küreselleşmenin öteki yüzü: yoksulluk* (Other face of globalization: Poverty). İstanbul: İletişim Yayinlari.

Turkish Demographic and Health Survey-TDHS. (2005). *Türkiye Nüfus ve Sağlık Araştırması-*2003. Ankara: Hacettepe University Population Studies Institute.

Turkish Statistical Institute-Turkstat. (2006). Accessed October 28, 2009, from http://www.tuik.gov.tr/PreHaberBultenleri.do?id=482&tb_id=1

Turkish Statistical Institute-Turkstat. (2007). *Household labour survey 2007*. Accessed October 28, 2009, from www.turkstsat. gov.tr/Pre/statistiktablo.do?istab_id=542

Turkish Statistical Institute-Turkstat. (2007a). Accessed September 29, 2008, from http://www.tuik.gov.tr/PreHaberBultenleri.do?id=626&tb_id=1

UNDP. (2001). *Measuring Turkey's HD performance*. Accessed November 1, 2009, from www.un.org/tr/undp/pdf/nhdr/ozet/pdf

UNDP. (2004). *Human development report: Information and communication technologies*. Accessed November 3, 2009, from www.undp.org.tr/publicationsDocumentsNHDR2004eng final.pdf

UNICEF-IRC (2005). *Child poverty in rich countries*. Florence: Author.

World Bank. (2000). *Turkey economic reforms, living standards and social welfare study*. (Report No. 20029-TU). Washington, DC: Author.

World Bank (2003). *Turkey, poverty and coping after crisis*. Washington, DC: Author.

World Bank. (2005). *Turkey education sector study*. (Report No: 32450-TU). Washington, DC: World Bank.

Roma Children and Social Exclusion in Lithuania: Sociological Approach to Human Development

Tadas Leončikas and Vida Beresneviciute

1 Roma in Lithuania: Baseline Situation

Census data in 2001 identified 2,571 persons who declared their ethnicity as Gypsy or Roma in Lithuania (Statistics Lithuania (2002)).[1] However, it is estimated that there may actually be up to 3,000 Roma (HRMI, 2005), because the census may not have reached a substantial part of the Roma in problematic neighbourhoods and may also have underreported the real number because of Roma working abroad. Although most Roma in the Baltic countries are sedentary,[2] they participated in the large emigration waves from the Baltic countries throughout the 1990s and since 2000, and their population may have decreased somewhat by now even if the afore-mentioned estimation was correct. Many Roma, usually with families, have moved to Great Britain since 2000, which is one of the most important labour migration destinations for Lithuanians in general. The Roma returnees report their positive labour experiences (emphasizing that their ethnic background was of little importance to their employers or colleagues in Britain), and this contrasts sharply with the massive unemployment of Roma in their countries of origin. Such experience presents a good counter-argument to those who believe that there are certain elements in "Roma culture" that discourage Roma from employment. In 2008, more than one-half of the surveyed Lithuanian Roma (52%) had a family member or someone from their close social environment living abroad at the time of the survey.

Although the Roma group in Lithuania may look small in comparison to the large proportions of the population in Central European states or even in neighbouring Latvia, the Lithuanian case shows clearly that the extent of problems experienced by

T. Leončikas (✉)
Centre of Ethnic Studies, Institute for Social Research, Vilnius LT-08105, Lithuania
e-mail: leoncikas@ktl.mii.lt

[1] For a comparison, see the figures in other Baltic countries: the census registered 8,204 Roma in Latvia (2000), and 542 in Estonia (2000) (Statistics Latvia (2002); Public database of Statistics Estonia).

[2] Many research papers contain a repeated reference to the 1956 decree of the Supreme Council of the USSR that required the nomadic Roma to register and get employed.

S. Andresen et al. (eds.), *Children and the Good Life*, Children's Well-Being: Indicators and Research 4, DOI 10.1007/978-90-481-9219-9_14, © Springer Science+Business Media B.V. 2010

a minority is not related to its size. Due to social isolation, Roma in Lithuania may have retained somewhat more features of traditional communal structures and customs than Roma populations affected more strongly by modernization. For instance, it is common for Roma groups in Lithuania to speak their variant of Romanes as their mother tongue; linguistic assimilation is not observed. However, isolation is also being reproduced by their social exclusion in contemporary society, with one outcome being a lack of educated Roma and therefore a lack of community representation. In comparison to Roma in other countries, there is a notable lack of successful Roma NGOs and a lack of examples of public careers by Roma representatives in Lithuania.

2 Roma and Public Education System

Although detailed demographic studies of Roma are lacking, the last census data reveal a prevalence of young people among the Roma: 46% of the Roma population in Lithuania are under 20 years and 35.5% are under 15 years of age (see Figs. 1 and 2); in Latvia, 27% are under 15.[3,4] However, the proportions may not be entirely representative due to inaccuracies during the census, as Roma children may have been easier to register than some mobile adults. Therefore, this data could be viewed as sufficient for planning educational assistance, but should not be used to reinforce simplistic stereotypes about Roma reproduction patterns. In fact, survey data reveal that Roma family size in the Baltic countries is not so unusual, even if it differs from the ageing mainstream population: An average Roma family size in Latvia in 2000 was 4.2 persons (in comparison to the Latvian average of 2.8); the average number of children in Roma families in Lithuania was 2.4.[5] These figures, nonetheless, mean that a major population subgroup suffering from massive exclusion from the labour market and the public education system[6] is of a relatively young age. Therefore, one can predict that this ethnic group is likely to remain confined within the reproduction of poverty if no structural changes occur.

---

[3]This chapter is based on previous work covering various aspects of educational issues: HRMI (2005); Leončikas (2006, 2009); "Developments of Roma community in the Baltics" in GESIS Social Science Thematic Series.

[4]Calculated on the basis of data provided in Leončikas (2006) and Statistics Latvia (2002) Latvijas 2000 gada tautas skaitišanas rezultati [Results of the 2000 National Census in Latvia]. Riga: Centrala statistikas parvalde.

[5]Data come from Latvian Centre for Human Rights and Ethnic Studies (2003, p. 17) and from a 2007 survey of Lithuanian Roma (N = 119), reported in Centre of Ethnic Studies, 2007. In the latter case, the average number of children was calculated on the basis of only those respondents who have children.

[6]With regard to continuing deprivation of Roma population in these policy areas, see the periodic reports on the Baltic countries by the European Commission against Racism and Intolerance (ECRI).

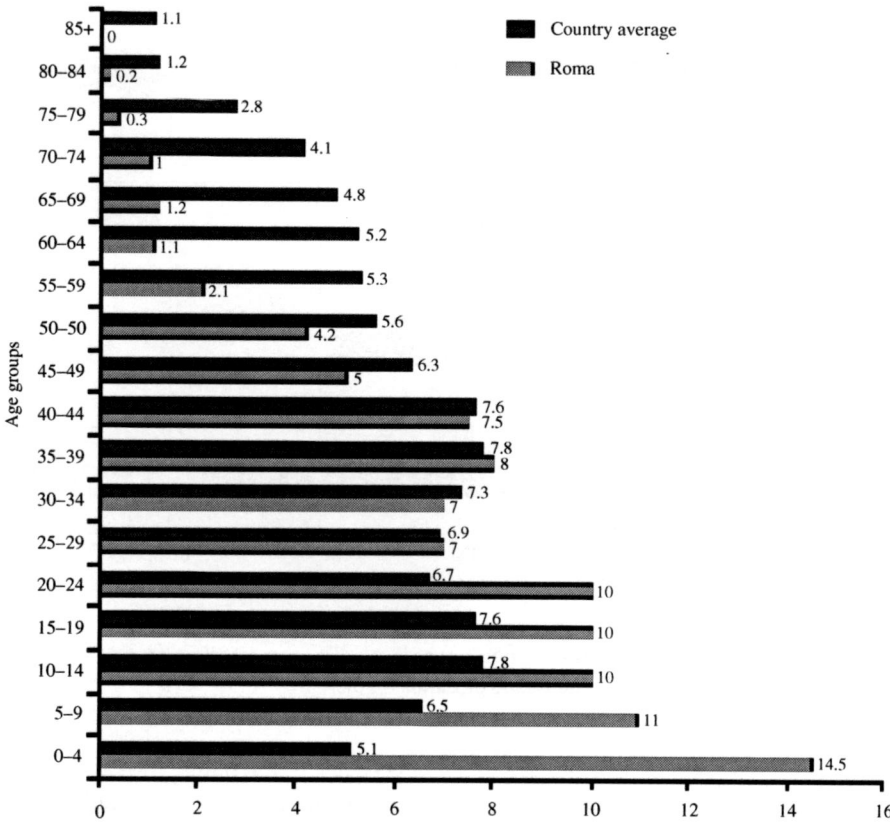

Fig. 1 Roma age structure and country average (according to 2001 census data)

A detailed analysis of 2001 Lithuanian census data reveals that the younger Roma generation knows less of the Lithuanian language than the older age groups. Within the main socially active age group of 20–39-year-olds, over 30% of Roma stated that they do not know Lithuanian (38% was the overall rate; the highest percentage was among the youngest respondents). In comparison to other ethnic groups, Roma have one of the largest proportions of persons with no knowledge of the state language. Moreover, there is a "regressive tendency" with respect to age. According to Lithuanian census data, more members of young generations of ethnic minorities speak the state language than older ones. The contrary trend, that is, regressive knowledge of the state language among the Roma, shows that their isolation and exclusion have increased. This is probably an indicator that the young generation has less out-group contact within the surrounding social environment and within the educational system than it used to do in the Soviet past.

Needless to say, the language barrier may additionally aggravate the educational development of the Roma community as well as their opportunities to acquire qualifications, participate in training courses or find a job (HRMI, 2005, p. 13). On the

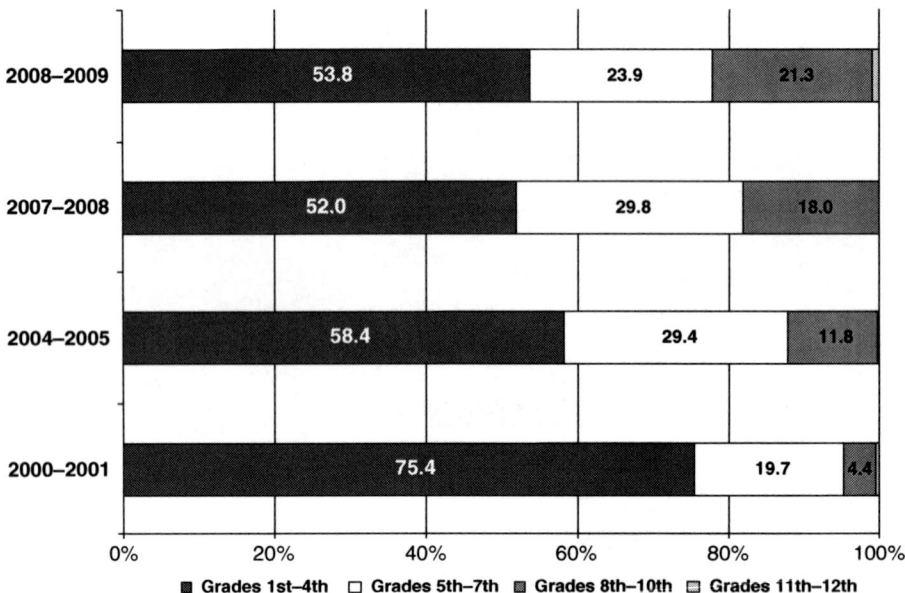

Fig. 2 Distribution of Roma children by grades attended in the school years 2001–2008 (per cent) Sources: Data on 2000–2001 and 2004–2005 from the Foundation for Educational Change; 2007–2008 and 2008–2009 from the Centre of Ethnic Studies

other hand, the peculiar sensitivity to language issues in the public discourse in the Baltic countries tends to hide the fact that many undereducated Roma could potentially work in those labour market sectors where linguistic competencies are not essential (unqualified work sectors), and that they are excluded on the basis of their ethnicity and not on the basis of their knowledge of languages.

Roma enrolment both in schools with instruction in the state language and in schools with minority (Russian) language has been increasing slightly since 2000 with the overall number of students reaching 579 in 2008 (Centre of Ethnic Studies, 2008).[7] However, regardless of whether the second language of Roma is a state or minority language, school attendance is low, dropout rates are high and late start of school education (e.g. entrance to 1st grade only at the age of 10) is common.[8]

Factors affecting inclusion into the education system are closely related to a set of interdependent social circumstances that limit the development and formalisation of social skills, access to social opportunities and their application for the purposes

---

[7] The educational expert V. Toleikis has suggested that Roma, who have a generally low knowledge of the mainstream (state) language, encounter a double barrier of integration when they have to adapt to a minority social milieu and then also overcome a state language barrier.

[8] For factual descriptions, see the 2005 report of the European Monitoring Centre on Racism and Xenophobia "Roma and Travellers in Public Education" (Vienna), and the corresponding country reports on which it is based.

of social integration. The survey of Lithuanian Roma showed that despite a slight increase in the number of Roma continuing education beyond primary level, most do not even acquire basic education. Basic and secondary (i.e. post-primary stages of) education remain a challenge. Estimates on the ages of starting and finishing school reveal that, on average, the surveyed Roma attended school for 6–7 years and completed five grades. However, a major proportion of young Lithuanian Roma (one-third of those below 18 years) started school at the age of 10 or later (Centre of Ethnic Studies, 2008). Nonetheless, analyses of the data from the last decade show some positive developments despite the major concentrations of Roma pupils at the primary level of education. In 2008, the distribution among other levels of secondary education was increasing (see Fig. 2). To view the educational attainment data in a broader perspective, it must be noted that at the community level, there are no signs of social advancement: Over one-half of the Lithuanian Roma (2008 survey) have not acquired a higher education level than their parents. It is also notable that little change has occurred on the family level either: Late starters often come from families in which parents began attending school later than the usual age (Centre of Ethnic Studies, 2008). It also means that neither social workers nor representatives of the educational system manage to notice these situations and make timely interventions.

One innovation that could have exerted some influence was the introduction of preschool classes at the Roma Community Centre established in the impoverished Roma settlement in Kirtimai district of Vilnius in 2002.[9] In contrast to warnings about the risk of segregation from international observers such as the ECRI (European Commission against Racism and Intolerance) or the European Roma Rights Centre, experiences with Roma-only preschool preparatory classes have been rather positive, because the children then became more ready to successfully enter 1st-grade primary school. However, regardless of positive experiences or of lessons that could be learned from problematic experiences, it is still difficult to grant Roma educational measures sufficient policy priority to make them more systematic.[10]

3 Social Context of Children's Experiences

One of the particular social context dimensions that makes it difficult to target policy on the disadvantaged Roma population is a nearly universal popular belief that the Roma have chosen their way of life themselves. In the media, Roma are associated almost exclusively with news on crime and the drug trade.

---

[9]Examples include classes in Ventspils (Latvia) or Kirtimai Roma Community Centre (Vilnius, Lithuania), where specially trained and/or assisted teachers work (see: Latvian Centre for Human Rights and Ethnic Studies, 2003, p. 23; Leončikas, 2006, p. 112).

[10]The attempts to involve Roma mediators or teacher assistants in Latvia and Lithuania were project-based. Even when supported through governmental funds (such as Roma integration programme in Lithuania), they did not result in systemic assistance to Roma. For more information on this type of measure, see Rus (2006).

Against this background, the Roma have remained the most disliked ethnic group in Lithuania over the last few years. Data from attitude surveys in 2009 show that the majority of the Lithuanian population would not like to have Roma as their neighbours (58%), as co-workers (50%) or as housing tenants (76%). The regular measurements of social distance (as evidenced by the negative attitude towards accepting certain groups as neighbours) reveal that even when the general level of intolerance is changing, the hierarchy of disliked groups remains the same with the Roma at the top. In fact, the Roma tend to be associated with and evaluated as a problematic social group rather than as an ethnic or cultural group. In public awareness, Roma fall into one cluster with such categories as ex-prisoners, drug addicts and alcohol addicts, and not with other ethnic groups.[11] With this poor informational background, the negative attitude prevails not only in the media, but also among policymakers, schools, or, for example, the parents of children attending mainstream schools who become concerned if Roma from impoverished environments come to the same school as their offspring (Fig. 3).

The public image of Roma is actually determined by exaggerated representations of the crime problems in the Kirtimai, the largest concentrated Roma settlement in the Baltic countries situated in the industrial area of Vilnius. It has around 500 inhabitants and nearly 100 wooden buildings in which substandard living conditions prevail and basic amenities such as water or sanitation are lacking. City authorities persistently refuse to enter any compromise regarding a possible legitimisation of

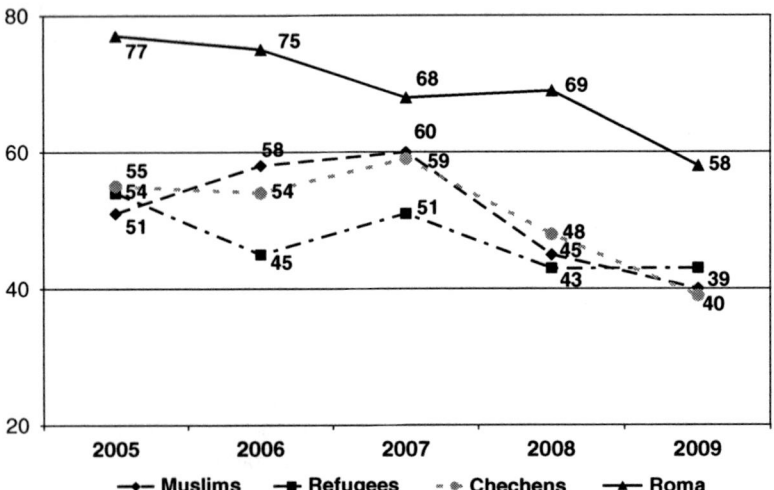

Fig. 3 Which groups would you not like to have as your neighbours? 2005–2009 (percent) Source: Centre of Ethnic Studies (http://www.ces.lt). Note: Selected examples from a large list are presented in this graph for comparison

[11] This statement is based on factor analysis of the item "Whom you would not like to have as your neighbours?" from the 1999 European Values Survey data from Lithuania (Leončikas, 2007).

the settlement, and they demolished six buildings in 2004 at the peak of a municipal campaign to curtail drug trade in the settlement. Nonetheless, municipal campaigns to introduce law and order were short-lived, and the drug trade in the settlement remains pervasive. However, instead of taking the complex approach to community development that is necessary in the de facto ghettoised settlement, the media reinforce only a superficial criticism of Roma as the willing perpetrators of the drug trade.

When children and their socialization are taken into consideration, it becomes clearer that this is not a social environment that has been chosen voluntarily. Even though Roma live in varying conditions aecross the country, the settlement in Kirtimai requires special attention due to the degree of social ostracism. Morally judged and both socially and geographically excluded, any inhabitant in Kirtimai carries a burden of societal condemnation that is applied collectively. This contemporary practice of collective responsibility is also hitting children through a popular belief that the family is the primary unit responsible for the child's preparation for schooling and so forth. This logic leads to the idea that when Kirtimai children drop out of school, it is their own problem or the responsibility of the families and not a failure of the educational agencies or a matter of social policy. The general policy schemes seem to be ineffective in targeting the small, but disadvantaged young Roma population.

The Roma settlement as a danger to society is a popular topic in the media that provides a flow of negative information on and criminalizes associations with the Roma community. When portraying children, there is a lack of attention to protecting the child's privacy and well-being. One example is a report on Kirtimai in a popular journal *Panele* (2008) for youngsters, in which photos of Roma youngsters (under age of 18) were followed by accounts of their intimate experiences without a proper review before publishing.

In the framework of the National Report on Strategies of Lithuania for Social Protection and Social Inclusion 2006–2008,[12] Lithuania has chosen the following priorities: increasing labour market participation, improving access to quality services, eliminating child poverty[13] and tackling disadvantage in education and training. The last two should have targeted the children's situation. According to

---

[12]National report on strategies of Lithuania for social protection and social Inclusion 2006–2008 with the annexe Tasks and Measures in Reducing Poverty and Social Exclusion. http://ec.europa.eu/employment_social/social_inclusion/docs/2006/nap/lithuania_en.pdf

[13] According to statistics, the at-risk-of-poverty rate is higher among children than among other age groups, and Lithuanian children are the social group with the highest poverty-risk rate. According to Statistics Lithuania, those at risk of poverty are mostly persons living in households with a single adult and dependent children (48.3%), two adults with three and more children (46.0%) and single persons (47.7%). Compared to 2007, the risk of poverty for persons living in large families (households with two adults and three and more children) increased by 7.2 percentage points and by 6.8 percentage points for those living in one-parent families (households consisting of one adult and dependent children). A large share of income of persons living in one-parent families consisted of alimony, support from relatives and social transfers; whereas in 2007, the increase in this income was less than that in earned income. See: *Statistics Lithuania.* Income

experts, the policy priorities in Lithuania have been limited to the childcare approach associated mainly with the "material situation", and ignore other important dimensions of child well-being such as subjective well-being, children's relationships, civic participation, risk and safety (Poviliunas, 2007). In general, the institutional framework in Lithuania lacks any focus on preventive measures against child poverty. Roma children fall under the supervision of different institutional measures, and there is a lack of any assessment of the individual needs of a child. One example of a targeted approach is an initiative of the Children's Rights Ombudsman Institution of the Republic of Lithuania, a child's rights monitoring and control governmental institution. In 2004, it initiated evaluation of children's situations in the Roma settlement of Kirtimai. The main emphasis of the evaluation was on the drug trade as a damaging environment for children. In this context, Roma children are much more affected by the general exclusion of Roma than by any social policy measures. In other words, the primary social status of the Roma child in Lithuanian society is Roma, not child. In the case of the Roma, the educational system also contributes to the reproduction of social exclusion and poverty.

The social outcomes of the aforementioned statements can be uncovered by analysing the dynamics of these processes with a focus on the life course. Comparisons of some available indicators can be made between Roma and the national average. They define a biographical trajectory of a Roma, and enable us to elaborate on their multilevel disadvantages (see Table 1). Acquisition of a driving licence is one illustrative example of how weak education and illiteracy place Roma at a disadvantage when it comes to formalising social skills and exercising them for social integration.

However, there may be good grounds for arguing that a focus on children's rights is not sufficient for promoting social change, and that more attention should be given to the social background and biographical prospects of the new generation of Roma. Social changes observed in the Roma community reveal new issues requiring targeted attention. As mentioned above, the 2001 census revealed that Roma youth have less knowledge of the Lithuanian language than older generations, and this leads to greater social isolation. Changes in family structures among the Roma (e.g. family break ups, at-risk families, migration), occasional reports on abandoned Roma children or problems with foster parents exert a significant influence on Roma children. Even in the period of rapid economic growth and low unemployment, there had been no support mechanisms for Roma youth to enter the labour market or to return to the educational institutions. The previously known problem of the drug trade in the Roma community is bringing new troublesome outcomes. Previously, Roma were mainly dealing in drugs without using them themselves; now the number of drug users is increasing rapidly and spreading to the younger generations as well.

---

and living conditions of the population, risk of poverty. Press Release, 16.10.2009. Available at: http://www.stat.gov.lt/en/news/view/?id=7602.

Table 1 Biographical trajectory of a Roma

		Roma[a]	National average
Entrance into education	Preschool (children)	30.7%	71.7%[b]
	Primary (retrospective data for Roma)	28.1%	92.8%[c]
	Basic (retrospective data for Roma)	22.1%	94.9%[d]
Duration of education	Starting schooling at age of (years old)	7.6 (adults) 6.9 (children)[e]	6
	Estimated duration of schooling (years)	6.8 (adults) ~ 7 (children)	10.0 (among 7–16 years-olds)[f]
Household, family		*Roma[g]*	*National average*
	Birth of first child at age of (years)	20	25[h]
	Number of children	3.67	1.25[i]
	Average size of household	6.5	2.4[j]
Household, family (continued)	First marriage at age of (years)	No data/Majority not registered	Women: 25 Men: 27[k]
	Departure from family home at age of (years)	Women: 18 Men: 17.3	
	Number of marriages (partnerships)	78.4% living in their first marriage (either registered or not)	Nearly 50% divorced[l]

Table 1 (continued)

	Roma[a]	National average
Social housing	30.8% in municipal housing	Social housing makes 2.4%[m] of total households
Driving		
Driver's licence obtained at age of (in years)	24.5 (those above 30); 17.2% of those under 30 have a license (youngest - 23)	Average age of applicants: 30 51% of those under 21 have a licence (2008)[n]
First car obtained at age of (years)	26.3	No data

[a]Source: Centre of Ethnic Studies, 2008

[b]Data for 2007: Mokymosi aprėptis pagal švietimo lygius. Švietimas 2007. Statistikos departamentas, Vilnius 2008. ISSN 1392-978X. 16 psl.

[c]Data for 2007: Mokymosi aprėptis pagal švietimo lygius. Švietimas 2007. Statistikos departamentas, Vilnius 2008. ISSN 1392-978X. 16 psl.

[d]Data for 2007: Mokymosi aprėptis pagal švietimo lygius. Švietimas 2007. Statistikos departamentas, Vilnius 2008. ISSN 1392-978X. 16 psl.

[e]Data from the Roma survey: adults indicated their age and children's age of the school start.

[f]Data for 2007 on presumptive duration of education of 7–16-year-old population. In 1997, this indicator equalled 9.9 years; since 1999, it has been stable—10 years; in the group of 7–18-year-olds—11.8 years. Source: Švietimas 2007. Statistikos departamentas, Vilnius 2008. ISSN 1392-978X. 17 psl.

[g]Source: Centre of Ethnic Studies, 2008.

[h]Lietuvos moterys 2006 metais. Statistinis portretas, 2007 03 07, http://www.stat.gov.lt/lt/ news/view/?id=1883.

[i]Lietuvos moterys 2006 metais. Statistinis portretas, 2007 03 07, http://www.stat.gov.lt/lt/ news/view/?id=1883.

[j]Lietuvos šeima šiandien, 2007 05 11, http://www.stat.gov.lt/lt/news/view/?id=2306.

[k]Lietuvos šeima šiandien, 2007 05 11, http://www.stat.gov.lt/lt/news/view/?id=2306.

[l]Lietuvos šeima šiandien, 2007 05 11, http://www.stat.gov.lt/lt/news/view/?id=2306.

[m]Lietuvos būsto strategija, 2004 01 23, http://www.am.lt/VI/article.php3?article_id=2282.

[n]Valstybės monė Regitra, Gausėja pradedančių vairuotoj* gretos, 2008 01 28; Dauguma pradedančių vairuotoj—moterys, 2008 09 17; Teisę vairuoti lengvuosius automobilius gijo 37 proc. daugiau gyventoj, 2008 07 16; http://www.regitra.lt/index.php?Action=Naujienos& Action1=Nauja_placiau&trump=ne.

Given the lack of policy measures aimed at young adults and the rarity of cooperation between different institutions, Roma youth in Lithuania caught between school and the labour market find themselves in the middle of nowhere. Roma leave the educational institutions at an early age with poorly developed personal, social, training and other skills and competencies; and, after several years, they disappear from any institutional records or measures of social support. Complaints made by Roma to specialised bodies such as the equal opportunity Ombudsperson (since 2004) or the Seimas Ombudsmen's Office of the Republic of Lithuania reveal attempts by Roma people to solve issues related first to housing followed by employment or social support, but not issues related to education or youth. The content of the complaints and their increase deliver a signal regarding the need for or failure of preventive mechanisms. Without developing this area of targeted policy, many other inputs are in vain and cannot bring about any generational change.

4 Roma Integration Policy Context

Educational and child-oriented projects have been the most substantial and most developed part of Roma integration policy in Lithuania since the 1990s. So why has there not been substantial change in Roma exclusion?

There is a strong conviction against a neoliberal background to the economy and policymaking that school attendance is merely an individual concern (or that of an individual family).[14] This is accompanied by a widespread lack of sensitivity towards deficiencies in the educational system, the absence of means for active inclusion and the incompetence of policymakers and educational bureaucrats when it comes to introducing measures to promote motivation (in our case, to encourage Roma pupils). This may be an outcome of a predominance of neoliberal approaches to policy that has prevailed since the 1990s and ignores the need to combine educational policies with social integration measures. The introduction of competitive mechanisms between schools with a school's funding depending on the number of pupils it attracts[15] has had ambiguous effects for the Roma: some schools enrol Roma into official lists to increase general funding and then keep silent when Roma children fail to attend school properly. Schools attracting pupils with a higher social profile discourage Roma enrolment and attendance in order not to scare off the mainstream parents. Education is the only single social institute that approaches the largest share of the Roma population at one time and could serve as means for networking and referral to other institutions, but the aforementioned issues have received surprisingly little critical analysis so far. Cooperation between different

---

[14]The situation in Lithuania is similar in this respect to that found in Latvia: "most officials and schoolteachers did not think that schools, local governments or the state should shoulder the responsibility for this situation. They expressed the view that the Roma themselves must deal with it" (Latvian Centre for Human Rights and Ethnic Studies, 2003, p. 23).

[15]The so-called pupil's basket principle, or "money follows a client".

social institutes remains a challenge for the Roma at different stages in their life courses because general policy measures (that target specific social groups such as the disabled, long-term unemployed, drug addicts, dropouts etc.) fail to consider a small group with very specific social needs.

Generally speaking, the research data and the reflections on policy contexts lead to the following conclusions on the most relevant aspects of Roma involvement in the educational system and also points to future challenges:

Poor school attendance and frequent dropout are related to delayed school enrolment (for example, at 10–11 *years).* The high dropout rate is generally credited as one of the major issues in Roma education. However, even temporary school attendance should be stressed as an important step. Early enrolment of children and purposeful support measures for Roma should be emphasized for their integration into the general education system.

Kindergarten and preschool education and regular support from social workers and special teachers help encourage better attendance, timely development of social skills, and learning.

The disproportionate number of Roma children attending specialized schools indirectly confirms that Roma needs are not met in general education schools. The specialized education system partially encourages Roma parents to enrol their children in specialised schools. Yet if the need for social support was satisfied in other ways, a certain percentage of school children who now attend specialized schools could be integrated into the general education system.

Studies reveal that a better understanding of the specific social and learning needs of Roma and working with them to meet these needs enables them to improve their situation within the general education system. To avoid Roma discrimination and segregation, more attention should be paid to identifying their individual needs instead of treating them as one general group that is associated with low education expectations and therefore having to meet relatively lower requirements. One of the educational challenges is to provide relevant support to teachers who work with Roma school children.

So far, general education schools have made little use of the experience gained by NGOs and other institutions working with Roma. A range of organizations and institutions are helping the Roma to cooperate both on the NGO level and with state institutions. However, organized and consistent changes need to be achieved.

The lack of progressive change in the Roma situation over the last two decades since the demise of the Soviet regime is in sharp contrast to the expectations of policymakers that a new generation of Roma will bring about change. On the contrary, we see a reproduction of poverty and exclusion. This chapter argues that the failure to provide social assistance through educational institutions and networks has been one of the main reasons for the growing marginalization of the Roma during the last decade. In order to develop a systemic policy approach, it is necessary to take a new look at the impact areas as well as indicators of problems and indicators of achievement.

References

Centre of Ethnic Studies. (2007). *Rom bendruomenės socialinės integracijos galimybi tyrimas* [Research on opportunities for social integration of Roma community]. Research commissioned by Lithuanian Office of the Equal Opportunities Ombudsperson. Accessed December 8, 2009, from http://www.lygybe.lt/ci.admin/Editor/assets/Romu%20integrac%20galimybes%20ataskaita.pdf

Centre of Ethnic Studies. (2008). *Rom padėties tyrimas: romai švietimo ir darbo rinkos sankirtoje* [Roma at the crossroads of the education and labour market]. Study commissioned by the Department of National Minorities and Lithuanians Living Abroad under the Government of the Republic of Lithuania.

Human Rights Monitoring Centre. (2005). *Roma: Situation assessment* (pp. 18–20). Accessed December 8, 2009, from http://www.hrmi.lt/downloads/structure//Romu_padeties_analize_20050412%20ENG121.pdf

Latvian Centre for Human Rights and Ethnic Studies. (2003). *The situation of Roma in Latvia*. Accessed December 28, 2009, from http://www.humanrights.org.lv/html/news/publications/roma_latvia.html

Leončikas, T. (2006). Rom švietimo iššūkiai [Challenges of Roma education]. *Ethnicity Studies, 1*, 87–120.

Leončikas, T. (2007). Nepakantumo hierarchija ir socialinė distancija visuomenės mažum atžvilgiu [Hierarchy of intolerance and social distance towards minorities]. In R. Žiliukaitė (Ed.), *Dabartinės Lietuvos kultūros raidos tendencijos: vertybiniai virsmai* (pp. 89–107). Vilnius: Kultūros, filosofijos ir meno institutas.

Leončikas, T. (2009). Developments of Roma community in the Baltics. In: GESIS Leibniz Institute for the Social Sciences (Ed.): *Roma in Central and Eastern Europe*. (pp. 44–51) Berlin: Gesis.

Poviliunas, A. (2007). *Lithuania. Tackling child poverty and promoting the social inclusion of children. A study of national policies. Peer review and assessment in social inclusion.* Accessed December 8, 2009, from http://ec.europa.eu/employment_social/spsi/docs/social_inclusion/experts_reports/lithuania_1_2007_en.pdf

Public database of Statistics Estonia. Accessed December 28, 2009, from http://www.stat.ee

Rus, C. (2006). The Situation of Roma School Mediators and Assistants in Europe. DGIV/EDU/ROM (2006) 3. Accessed August 1, 2010 from http://www.coe.int/t/dg4/education/roma/Source/Mediators_Analyse_EN.pdf

Statistics Latvia. (2002). *Latvijas 2000 gada tautas skaitišanas rezultati* [Results of the 2000 National Census in Latvia]. Riga: Centrala statistikas parvalde.

Statistics Lithuania. (2002). *Gyventojai pagal lyt, amži, tautybę ir tikybą* [Population by sex, age, ethnicity and religion]. Vilnius: Statistikos departamentas.

Index

S. Andresen et al. (eds.), *Children and the Good Life*, Children's Well-Being:
Indicators and Research 4, DOI 10.1007/978-90-481-9219-9,
© Springer Science+Business Media B.V. 2010

Lightning Source UK Ltd.
Milton Keynes UK
27 October 2010

161992UK00005B/25/P